Conducting Your Pharmacy
Practice Research Project

Conducting Your Pharmacy Practice Research Project

A step-by-step guide

Felicity J Smith

BPharm, MA, PhD, MRPharmS

Professor of Pharmacy Practice
School of Pharmacy
University of London, UK

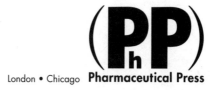

London • Chicago **Pharmaceutical Press**

Published by the Pharmaceutical Press
An imprint of RPS Publishing

1 Lambeth High Street, London SE1 7JN, UK
100 South Atkinson Road, Suite 206, Grayslake, Il 60030-7820, USA

© Pharmaceutical Press 2005

RPS Publishing is the wholly-owned publishing organisation of the
Royal Pharmaceutical Society of Great Britain

Reprinted 2006

Typeset by Photoprint, Torquay, Devon
Printed in Great Britain by TJ International Ltd, Padstow, Cornwall

ISBN-10 0 85369 606 3
ISBN-13 978 0 85369 606 3

Keele
University

Keele University Library - Checkout(s)
01782 733230

Customer ID: 14028691102

Title: Conducting your pharmacy practice
research project : a step-by-step guide /
ID: 6090902**68

Due: 06 March 2018

Total items: 1
20/02/2018 16:47

Please retain your receipt
http://keele-primo.hosted.exlibrisgroup.com

Contents

Preface

The scope of pharmacy practice research is huge. This is a reflection of the fact that, in order to promote safe and appropriate drug use, pharmacists have to take so many issues into account. New directions in health policy, changing needs and expectations of the population, the structural, economic, social and cultural contexts of healthcare, and the aspirations of pharmacists for a greater role in its delivery all provide the background and frameworks for the conception and execution of pharmacy practice research. Equally diverse is the range of approaches and methods that may be employed to answer important questions.

A further attraction of the discipline is its value. The research is rarely undertaken out of curiosity but with a particular end or application in view. Pharmacy practice research is important to patients, healthcare organisations, governments and the profession. The ultimate goal is to lead the way in the adaptation of pharmacy services to meet health and pharmaceutical care needs and contribute to pharmacy and health policy agendas.

Participation in original research is also seen as a fundamental component in the education of students. The Royal Pharmaceutical Society of Great Britain's accreditation requirements for a pharmacy degree and the Quality Assurance Agency for Higher Education's criteria for the award of a Master's degree include descriptors relating to the understanding of research methodology, the acquisition of research skills and their application to an individual research project. However, conducting a pharmacy practice research project should be seen as an opportunity not only to develop personal skills but also to undertake an original piece of work that has the potential to influence services of the future.

For project work undertaken by students the responsibilities for different aspects of the research will be shared with their supervisors. The role of the supervisor may vary between institutions and the level of support required by students will depend on their research experience and the complexity of the work. Although this text aims to cover all principal activities associated with conducting a pharmacy practice research project, some of these may have been attended to in advance. In particular, the obtaining of ethical approval to undertake the work is often not the responsibility of the student. Also, as project work is generally of limited duration, students may be involved only with certain (although important) aspects of the research, e.g. pilot work and the development of instruments, validation of techniques or data analysis.

This book is principally for first-time researchers, providing an overview of the whole process of undertaking research from initial planning through to the presentation of the final report. In my career, both in conducting my own research and in the supervision of students, I have become only too aware of the many potential pitfalls that can jeopardise the scientific validity or successful completion of a project. This book complements a previous volume (*Research Methods in Pharmacy Practice*), also from the Pharmaceutical Press, which provides an extensive and detailed description and critique of the application of health services research methodology to studies in pharmacy settings.

Conducting research is a varied and challenging task. The work must be done well. But I hope it will not appear too daunting. If future developments in pharmacy services are to be beneficial to all concerned, they must be supported and informed by a secure research base.

Felicity Smith
April 2005

About the author

Felicity Smith is a registered pharmacist with experience of hospital and community pharmacy. After completing her PhD, evaluating the contribution of community pharmacists to primary healthcare in London, at the Department of General Practice and Primary Care, St Bartholomew's Hospital Medical College in London, Dr Smith joined the academic staff of the School of Pharmacy, University of London. She is currently a Professor in its Department of Practice and Policy. Felicity Smith is experienced in the application of a wide range of health services research methodologies and tools in pharmacy settings. Throughout her career she has remained actively involved in conducting and supervising research projects into many aspects of pharmacy services and drug use. She has authored a complementary text, *Research Methods in Pharmacy Practice*, also from the Pharmaceutical Press. This comprises a detailed review of published research undertaken in pharmacy and related settings, focusing on the application of health services research methodologies to this work. It identifies the particular challenges of pharmacy practice research and describes how potential problems have been, and can be, addressed.

1

The preparation and planning stages

Medicines are the core of healthcare, and thus pharmacy services should be central to their provision. Throughout the world, the organisation and delivery of healthcare are high on governments' agendas. The ever-evolving health policies, priorities and needs present new opportunities and challenges for pharmacy. We must be prepared to review our practices critically and innovate to meet the changing public expectations and health policy objectives of health and pharmaceutical care.

Research into the practice of pharmacy and the use of medicines is a branch of health services research that has become a huge industry. All health professionals have to be accountable for the care that they provide and demonstrate the worth of their services. As pharmacists, we need to show that our services, existing and new, are relevant to real healthcare needs, effective, of high quality, and continually being developed with wider health policy goals in mind.

Researchers from pharmacy, medicine, epidemiology, sociology, anthropology, psychology, history and economics, among others, have applied themselves to studies of pharmacy services and the use of medicines. This has stimulated many within the discipline of pharmacy to incorporate different approaches and methods into addressing pharmacy-related problems. Collaboration between pharmacists, other health professionals, voluntary organisations, consumers and/or members of the public is also a common feature of this research.

Thus, pharmacy practice research has a wide scope, drawing on methodologies of different disciplines and addressing complex problems in health and healthcare from a range of perspectives and settings. It is a challenging and exciting discipline. Conducting a pharmacy practice research project provides an opportunity to participate in the generation of new knowledge and contribute to the development of pharmacy services.

This chapter discusses the preparatory work and planning that takes place at the start of any study. This groundwork should be thorough. Time and care in these early stages enable the selection of appropriate design, methods and measures, which are essential for ensuring that the work is scientifically robust. Most studies are time limited. Awareness of the tasks that must be undertaken at the start (in particular those such as securing ethical approval, which must be achieved before the start of any fieldwork) is important in enabling realistic time planning and successful completion of the work.

This chapter discusses the following topics: literature review and preliminary fieldwork, specifying the aims and objectives, ethical approval and research governance, pilot studies, project management, conduct and a professional approach, and working with others.

LITERATURE REVIEW AND PRELIMINARY FIELDWORK

The literature review is generally the first task to be commenced, although the literature work and preliminary fieldwork are often concurrent. Together they provide a background for the study, in terms of identifying key issues to be addressed, devising and refining the aims and objectives of the study and selecting the most appropriate methods for the study. The literature review and preliminary fieldwork together lead to the development of the research protocol. The *research protocol* usually comprises the following:

○ Introduction and objectives: a statement of the aims and objectives of the research, together with some background to explain how they build on existing knowledge, meet an identified need and/or contribute to service development.

○ Methodology: explanation of the approach, methods and procedures with some justification for their selection and comments on how potential problems will be addressed. Separate sections may include details of sampling procedures, recruitment of participants, methods of data collection, research instruments and other documentation (e.g. questionnaires, data collection forms, information leaflets, consent forms, etc.) and proposals for the processing and analysis of data.

○ Details of the programme of work: including time scales, project milestones, management processes and anticipated outcomes.

New research should build on previous findings and take into account factors that are already known or thought to be important to the subject of study, i.e. not reinvent the wheel. A review of the literature focuses on previous research in the subject area, thus providing researchers with an insight into what is already known about a topic and relevant factors to take into account in their own work. There may also be issues pertinent to your work that have not been formally investigated by researchers, but have been reported anecdotally as important. Depending on the plausibility of these claims, you may wish to incorporate them. In terms of methodology, previous researchers may have devised and tested ways of collecting data or measuring important variables that could be usefully applied in your work. It is, of course, important to acknowledge your sources fully to avoid risks of plagiarism.

Preliminary fieldwork enables the researcher to ensure that the important issues from the perspective of the population of interest are identified. Thus, if the goal of the research is to assess the value of a new service from the perspective of health professionals and/or clients, the researcher may at the start have some informal discussions with a few key individuals to gain some insights into their expectations and experiences. This would ensure that issues important to these stakeholders could be incorporated when developing the protocol.

The literature review

A review of the literature is often a first major task of any research project. This aids in the development of the aims and objectives of the study and in devising a suitable methodology for meeting the objectives. A comprehensive literature review:

○   is important to ensure that the work builds on existing knowledge in the field, i.e. does not duplicate the work of others but builds on and extends this knowledge

○   allows the identification of factors that have been found by other researchers to be important to the topic or issues under study, so they can be taken into account

○   enables the identification of the perspectives of different stakeholders, so they can be addressed

○   assists in selecting the best methods for the study. There may be a number of ways of obtaining data relevant to the study objectives, all of which will have their strengths and weaknesses. Review of the methods used by others enables you to consider different options, together with their advantages and disadvantages, when planning your own work.

Finding relevant material

The literature review should be as comprehensive as possible. You want to avoid a situation in which relevant work is missed that would have been valuable in informing your study objectives. In pharmacy practice research this can be problem because of the interdisciplinary nature of many studies. Frequently, issues relevant to the study objectives may relate to professional practice, clinical issues and problems, and/or social science perspectives. These issues may have been addressed by researchers from different health professions, e.g. nursing, medicine and others as well as pharmacy, or from different academic disciplines, e.g. health psychology, epidemiology, sociology, etc. This may affect where the work is published and means that, in conducting the literature review, a wide range of databases, libraries and journals may have to be explored. As a result of the multidisciplinary and collaborative nature of much health service and pharmacy practice research, searching may have to extend to specialist clinical areas, social science databases, etc. Depending on the topic area, it can add to the value of a study if the possibility of contributions from other disciplines is considered. It may be worth keeping an open mind. Theoretical perspectives can provide an additional dimension to a research problem and sometimes a framework for the conceptualisation of a study.

In a systematic review of research, the selection of papers may be restricted to those that meet specific criteria, e.g. publication in a peer-reviewed journal or criteria relating to the scientific quality of the research. However, when developing a protocol for a research project, it may be appropriate to broaden the scope of the literature work to include material that, if not scientifically rigorous, still provides insights into relevant issues and perspectives for the topic of study. In healthcare research there will often be individuals and groups who have written about the problems that you are researching from their perspectives. Thus, in addition to research studies that are published in academic and professional journals, other types of document may be informative and valuable in planning the study. Thus, you may wish to include commentaries, e.g. by practitioners, researchers or other interested individuals, discussion articles written to promote debate, letters to journals, policy documents or material produced by various stakeholder groups. Special interest groups (professional and non-professional), government bodies and local health organisations may undertake research and/or produce documents representing their views and priorities. Exploration of a wide range of sources helps to ensure that the groundwork for the study is as comprehensive as possible.

Although computer databases are powerful and a valuable starting point, in most health service and pharmacy practice research some hand searching of journals is necessary. Not all journals in which relevant material may appear are included in databases of published research. In particular, articles in non-academic journals may be a useful source. It can also be difficult to ensure that all the necessary search terms have been identified. Commonly, a few key papers might be identified from a database, which provide a lead for further searches. The contents and references cited in these may provide useful leads to further important work – the identification of authors (researchers) who have an interest in the field and/or other journals that provide a forum for relevant research or commentaries. Research on particular topics may be concentrated in particular journals. Thus, after a database search you may target the contents/abstracts pages of these journals (which may be available online) to identify other relevant work.

However narrow or broad, the literature review should be as systematic as possible. All procedures should be well documented, and the search strategy clearly described and justified. Records of all searches should be maintained, whether or not these are productive, and should include details of the databases used, search terms, years of publication, language, specific journals or authors, use of libraries, the internet, etc. In addition, in relation to all relevant material, the full reference should be recorded (see Chapter 6 for details). It can be frustrating in the final stages of the work to discover that some of your references are incomplete or that you cannot remember the source of a particular piece of information.

Critical appraisal

When reviewing research papers, the findings and conclusions of a study must be interpreted in the context of the methods used. In terms of methodology, all studies will have their strengths and weaknesses. Compromises are often inevitable and they arise for all sorts of reasons, such as limited time or resources, ethical constraints, low response rates, poor judgement on the part of researchers or unforeseen difficulties that arise in the execution of the study. *Critical appraisal* is an important component of any review of the literature. You should reflect on the study design, sampling procedures, methods, instruments, measures, analytical processes, issues of reliability and validity, etc. You will then be in a position to consider the extent to which you think the study is of value and the conclusions are justified.

Preliminary fieldwork

The preliminary fieldwork, along with the literature review, informs the development of the study objectives and methodology. It:

○   assesses the importance of the research to various potential stakeholders and ensures that all their thoughts and concerns are identified and taken into account in designing the work

○   assists in the refinement of the aims and objectives

○   allows an exploration of the feasibility of different methodological approaches from the perspective of potential participants

○   informs the development of the research instruments

○   aids the preparation and review of documentation (information leaflets, data collection forms, etc.).

Preliminary fieldwork frequently involves informal discussions with interested parties, potential participants or their representatives. The aims will be, first, to ensure that the study objectives address the perspectives of these different groups and, second, that the methods and procedures of the study will be acceptable and workable. Preliminary fieldwork is sometimes designed to provide specific information required for the development of the research protocol, e.g. for a study involving hospital staff or patients you may need to find information on the number of staff or size of hospital. Preliminary fieldwork can be invaluable for the ultimate success of a research study. Discussing your proposal with interested individuals, who may have direct experience of the issues and problems and practicalities of conducting research in a particular setting, can be immensely helpful, improving your awareness of the subject area and the potential problems.

SPECIFYING THE AIMS AND OBJECTIVES

The aims of a study are generally more global statements, whereas the objectives are specific and measurable – they describe how the aim is to be achieved. The importance of having a clear statement of the aims and objectives cannot be underestimated. The objectives determine the design of the study (e.g. whether it is experimental or descriptive), the type of sample that is needed, the data that will be required and the analytical procedures necessary to answer precise questions. Precision in the objectives is vital to all stages of the work. A lack of clarity can result in an unfocused study that does not answer any research questions effectively.

The following is an example of a study's aim and objectives:

O   Study aim: to evaluate the effectiveness of a new pharmacy service.

O   Specific objectives may be to:

—   assess the feasibility of offering the service in a pharmacy setting, in terms of its acceptability to staff and consumers

—   estimate the time and costs involved in its operation

—   establish the knowledge and skills required by the people offering the service

—   measure the extent to which clinical outcomes are achieved

—   investigate clients' satisfaction with the service compared with existing care (such as time, accessibility, approachability of staff, the extent to which perceived needs are met, etc.).

Once precise objectives have been specified, you are then in a position to identify or devise suitable outcome measures for each. Think about each objective independently. How will it be addressed? In many cases, the literature will provide a useful source of possible approaches, methods and measures. If this is the case, these are often more robust than trying to devise your own. Otherwise, in a project that has a short timescale, you could end up spending most of the time developing and validating your methods and measures, leaving insufficient time for the main body of the work. In an experimental study the aim may be expressed as a hypothesis, e.g. that a new service will improve patient care. Objectives may then relate to assessment of the components of patient care, e.g. accessibility of professionals, quality of advice or clinical outcome. The study would be designed to test this hypothesis, and measures selected to assess the anticipated improvements (as expressed in the objectives).

In planning a study it is common to overestimate the amount that can be accomplished within a limited time. In health service and pharmacy practice research you are often dependent on other people to participate. You will have to fit in with their other commitments and work to their convenience. A tight data collection schedule may be unworkable in practice. There may be periods during the project when progress is slow. In particular, the time taken to arrange meetings for preliminary discussions, obtain ethical approval, recruit participants and await the return of questionnaires is a factor over which you have only limited control. Thus, in addition to being detailed and clear, the objectives must be realistically achievable. Attempting to meet too many objectives may be at the expense of addressing any of them properly.

A clear and precise statement of aims and objectives is important for:

○ the selection of a suitable study design

○ determining the most appropriate approach and methods so that all objectives are effectively addressed

○ development of the instruments: in particular ensuring that all the necessary information is gathered (with attention to its completeness, reliability and validity), while avoiding the collection of unnecessary data (which lengthens questionnaires or interviews and is inefficient)

○ providing a framework for analysis and appropriate procedures for meeting each objective.

ETHICAL APPROVAL AND RESEARCH GOVERNANCE

The Department of Health has published a research governance framework setting out broad principles for ensuring that healthcare and social care research is carried out to high scientific and ethical standards. The document discusses the roles and responsibilities of researchers, healthcare organisations and professionals in the research process. Healthcare organisations have responsibilities for the quality of care, including research activities. To comply with research governance principles and requirements, healthcare organisations have established their own procedures to ensure that standards are met. Thus, in addition to seeking ethical approval, researchers must also (preferably concurrently) apply to the relevant healthcare organisations and comply with their research governance procedures.

The research governance framework includes the requirement that research involving patients, service users, professionals and volunteers is reviewed independently to ensure that it meets ethical standards. High among these considerations is that the work respects the dignity, rights, safety and well-being of participants, and that the principle of informed consent is observed.

All research in the UK involving NHS staff, premises, facilities and patients must have approval from an NHS research ethics committee and each NHS trust in which the work is to take place. The Central Office for Research Ethics Committees (COREC) has been established to co-ordinate the development of standardised procedures and forms for the ethical review of healthcare research in the UK.

COREC recognises the special case of student projects (undergraduate and postgraduate) that would normally fall within the remit of NHS research ethics committees, but which are undertaken by students primarily for educational purposes. Separate procedures for review by student project ethics committees may apply.

An application to the research ethics committee will include all documentation relating to the study. The application form must be completed correctly and fully before the application will be considered. The research protocol describing the aims and objectives, all methods and procedures, including those to ensure the validity of data, will be required. Copies of the instruments (e.g. questionnaires, interview schedules, other data collection forms), information leaflets, consent forms, letters of recruitment, other documentation, etc. should also be included.

Ethical approval must be obtained before the start of the work. Therefore, applications for ethical approval must be undertaken well in advance of the planned starting dates of data collection.

All research raises ethical issues that must be addressed and these are wide ranging. When assessing the ethical implications an ethics committee will want to be satisfied of the ultimate value of the research, i.e. that it is worth doing. Research that requires the resources of the health service or the time of health professionals, and/or is a burden for potential participants, may be considered unethical if the findings are unlikely to be of value. Thus, the scientific validity of the research should be critically considered:

○ Are the design and methodology of the study appropriate and sufficiently robust to lead to valid results?

○ Are the anticipated findings likely to be relevant to the real needs of patients, health professionals and/or institutions, etc?

If these goals are unlikely to be met, then committing time and resources and compromising the convenience of others may not be justified.

Thus, in any application for ethical review, it is important to ensure that the relevance of the work, the expected value of the findings and the scientific validity of the research are clearly described. It should not be left to committee members to wonder about the value of the work. Other general issues to consider may be provision for involvement of people who speak other languages or attention to the special needs of particular groups.

Once the overall value of the research has been considered, you could then think about the methods and procedures of the research from the point of view of the potential participants:

○ What are you asking them to do? Are these requests reasonable?

○ Are you putting people to unnecessary risk or inconvenience?

○ Are the special needs of any particular groups identified and addressed?

If the work involves older people, children, or people who are sick or have other specific needs, guidance should be sought about additional considerations to safeguard their interests and rights. However worthy the goals of the research are, the dignity, rights, safety and well-being of participants are paramount.

In an ethical review, all aspects of the work should be critically considered so that potential concerns can be identified and addressed, e.g. with regard to specific proposals for recruitment and data collection in a pharmacy practice project, you may consider the following:

○ Are the procedures intrusive or too demanding? Are you expecting too much? Could the methods be modified?

O   Does an interview schedule include sensitive questions or explore topics that could be upsetting? If so, are you (and others involved in data collection) equipped to manage these situations?

O   Could the questions uncover concerns about the quality of care that a patient is receiving? If so, how will this be handled?

O   Could any of the questioning or observational procedures cause embarrassment? Will people be afforded sufficient privacy?

O   Could there be security concerns with regard to interviews conducted in people's own homes? If so, can you ensure that the interviewee is provided with information to identify the researcher in advance? The safety of the researchers must also be considered.

O   If you are employing others to assist with the data collection, how will you ensure that the research protocol will be closely followed by all?

The rights of the potential participants to the following must be respected:

O   Full information.

O   Genuine choice regarding participation.

O   Confidentiality of data.

Informed consent is central to research ethics. Participants should be fully informed as to what their participation will involve and how the data will be used, and should have opportunities to ask questions. Without this they will not be in a position to make an informed decision on whether or not to take part. Participants must feel free to make a choice and they should have time to consider their decision. They should also be assured that they are free to opt out at any time should they change their mind and that this would not affect their care or rights in any way.

Participants' rights to confidentiality must also be respected. Researchers will not have access to health or personal information of participants before obtaining their informed consent. Safeguards to ensure the confidentiality of data must be in place, e.g. consent forms with participants' names should be stored separately from the data, and only the members of the research team should have access to identity codes on questionnaires or other data collection documents. All data should be anonymised, names being omitted during the transcribing process.

Information leaflets should be prepared, possibly being distributed with letters inviting individuals to participate. These should explain to potential participants the purposes of the study, who is organising, funding and responsible for the work, and how and why particular people have been chosen to take part. Details of study procedures should be provided so that it is clear to people what will happen should they agree to take part. Potential participants should also be informed that their participation is voluntary, they are free to withdraw at any time, and all information will be kept strictly confidential and anonymised so that no one is identifiable in the results. Contact details should be provided so that people are able to seek further information. A proforma information sheet produced by the ethics committee may be suitable for adaptation for the study.

Written consent is generally required for all studies and must be obtained before the start of any data collection. The consent form often comprises a series of statements relating to the information and procedures of the project, with a space against each statement for participants to initial to indicate their understanding and/or consent. The form should be dated and signed by the participant and sometimes also by the person taking the consent. A proforma consent form may be available through the ethics committee or NHS organisation that can be adapted for your project.

No data collection can proceed until approval has been obtained from the appropriate ethics committee and NHS organisations. Although limited preliminary fieldwork (e.g. informal discussions with colleagues) will generally be undertaken before seeking ethical approval, more pilot work with potential research participants does not occur until approval is obtained. Thus, the timing of seeking ethical approval is important, and the process can be time-consuming and lengthy. It is important to plan ahead, to find out the exact requirements for the applications to these bodies and to prepare the documentation as soon as possible.

PILOT STUDIES

Pilot studies are conducted to test the methods, procedures, instruments and documentation of a study. If it is your study, you will want to be satisfied that these are working well, because this is essential for the success of the study. The pilot work provides you with the opportunity to make this assessment and identify and address any potential problems. After the pilot study you can review and modify the methods, procedures, instruments or other documentation. The purpose of a pilot study is twofold:

○ to check that the methods and procedures are acceptable and feasible in the research settings

○   to ensure that the chosen methods provide the data required (in terms of completeness, reliability and validity) to meet the study objectives.

In terms of study procedures and data collection, a pilot study should be a mini-version of the main study. However, the data analysis will be with the above objectives in mind, e.g. in a questionnaire or interview schedule you may look for inconsistencies in responses which may suggest ambiguity in the questions. Missing data may indicate that respondents had difficulty providing some information, or that there were some questions that were sensitive and which they did not want to answer.

You will want to look at the content of the data, e.g. did you obtain sufficient detail to enable you to address each study objective? Can you assess the extent to which the data provided were accurate? Did you receive any comments or feedback about other questions that you should include to ensure that you have a comprehensive picture of the issues that you are researching?

In relation to the acceptability of the process you may ask the following:

○   Were the recruitment rates good enough?

○   Were sufficient numbers of people eligible?

○   Were people prepared to take part?

○   If observing activities, could you be sufficiently discreet?

○   Did you find that your presence was a hindrance to others?

○   Was it possible to find a private area for interviewing?

The results of the pilot study may lead you to make some modifications to the study procedures, e.g.

○ modify the recruitment procedures, e.g. information provided to potential participants, or change the location of recruitment

○ reduce or extend a period of observation

○ amend an interview schedule, e.g. question order, reduce the length of an interview

○ rephrase questions in a questionnaire to ensure clarity

○ modify the layout of data collection form in an observation study

○ include additional questions on certain topics and/or omit others.

Even though the data obtained in the pilot work will probably not be included in the data-set for the main study, you should keep notes of the methods and procedures used, along with details of, and reasons for, any modifications made to the main study. Details of the pilot study should be included in the project report.

PROJECT MANAGEMENT: TIME SCALES AND
ADMINISTRATION

A time plan covering the duration of the project and including all stages of the work should be prepared at the start of the work. This will be helpful in enabling you to form an overview of the entire project. It should include all major tasks from the start until the presentation of the final report. It will also aid you in ensuring that enough time is allowed for each stage, identifying when you have less busy times, and in planning how these can be used productively. For example, while waiting for the return of questionnaires you could set up the data analysis file or start writing up the introduction, literature review and methodology for the final report.

Researchers are often over-ambitious regarding what can be achieved within a fixed time. It is important to be realistic when specifying objectives, and deciding on sample sizes and the amount of data to be collected. The time taken for some tasks is commonly underestimated. In particular, the preparation of applications to ethics committees and waiting for approval, recruitment of participants and receipt of completed questionnaires, and arranging interviews to suit the availability of others, are lengthy tasks over which you have only limited control. Following up non-responders to questionnaires, transcribing audio-recorded data, checking data for accuracy, and coding and analysing qualitative data sets can be very time-consuming.

Conducting a project requires good organisation. Throughout your project (from the start of your first ideas and reading), detailed notes should be kept of all your thoughts and decisions (with your reasoning) about how you will conduct the study. This should include careful records relating to the preparation of documentation, development of instruments, decisions about all aspects of study procedures, dealings with ethics committees, etc. These notes will be important in enabling you to justify your choice of methods.

A system should be devised to record details of all contacts relating to the project (personal, telephone, correspondence, etc.). It is very easy to forget which of your potential participants asked for more information, declined to participate, asked you to phone them back at a later date, were on holiday, etc. Notes should be made of any reasons given for non-response. Details of any difficulties experienced in the execution of the study may be helpful in enabling you to comment on the validity and any shortcomings in the study.

If other people are involved in the data collection or other stages of the work, you will also want to have systems in place for everyone to follow. This will also help you check the consistency with which procedures are applied and to ensure that there are formal opportunities for reporting and discussing any problems that arise. Problems in execution of the study should, of course, be addressed as soon as possible. Once the relevant stage of the project has passed, there will be no chance of modifying or clarifying procedures. Early recognition of, and attention to, problems will greatly enhance the accuracy, completeness and usefulness of the data.

CONDUCT AND A PROFESSIONAL APPROACH

People who take part in your research are doing you a favour. They will almost invariably have competing demands on their time, will usually derive no direct benefit and will agree to take part because they can see that the work may be of some future value. If you are a student they may see this value as limited to educational objectives. People will often be agreeable only if they can see that the work is relevant to some aspect of service development or patient care, carefully planned and professionally conducted, and that their rights are being observed. Although many studies depend on the goodwill of individuals, sometimes a nominal payment is made to participants in recognition of their time and expertise. This payment may also be to cover any expenses (e.g. travel) when these are not reimbursed separately.

Attention should be paid to maintaining a professional approach: good time keeping, appropriate self-presentation, adherence to agreed study procedures, and ensuring that the involvement of others is straightforward and procedures result in minimum inconvenience. As the researcher you must be willing to accommodate the commitments of participants (e.g. by arranging interviews at their convenience) and not expect them to fall in line. Forethought in ensuring that the procedures are workable in each setting will assist in the smooth operation and acceptability of the project, e.g. make sure that any need for access to a computer, power points, other facilities or documents will not hinder the work of staff, maintain a supply of spare batteries for recording equipment, etc. Throughout the work, it is the researcher who should 'do the running' and fit around the priorities and commitments of others, and not vice versa. An unprofessional approach could both jeopardise your work and discourage individuals from participating in future research.

Having taken part in a study, participants may like to be informed of the findings. It is good practice, after completion of the work, to send a letter of thanks and a summary of the findings (see Chapter 6) to everyone who was involved. If the work is published, a reprint can be sent. However, publication of research is generally a protracted process, usually at least one, and sometimes more than two, years from data collection. Participants should be informed of the planned progress of the study and when to expect information about the findings. A list of names and addresses of all participants and others who have assisted in the work or expressed an interest should be maintained and the information about the findings forwarded as soon as possible.

WORKING WITH OTHERS AND GROUP PROJECTS

Pharmacy practice research is almost invariably collaborative. At the very least, you are likely to require the cooperation of others during the data collection, e.g. as respondents to questionnaires, interviewees or hosts who agree to the presence of a researcher on their premises. Projects in health services research are commonly interdisciplinary and the contributions of people from different backgrounds and with particular skills and experience can be invaluable in ensuring that different perspectives are taken into account.

When working with others it is important to be clear from the start what the respective role and responsibilities of each person will be. For some projects, the level of involvement of different individuals will vary, e.g. some people may take responsibility for particular tasks or contribute expertise at a certain stage of the work. In other projects a group may work as a team, in which the levels of commitment of all members are expected to be similar and the responsibilities for all stages of the work are shared.

Some group projects fall naturally into a number of discrete parts. If this is so, each member of the team can take responsibility for one part, working more or less independently on this, albeit within an agreed broad framework. In other cases the team as a whole may be responsible for planning a project, developing a protocol, data collection, processing and analysis, and writing the final report. A team approach can confer a number of advantages. Ideas and expertise can be pooled. The objectives might be more ambitious, e.g. it may provide an opportunity to address a topic from a wider range of perspectives. It may be possible to extend sampling over a larger number of locations or to different groups of respondents. These features may enhance the relevance, generalisability and value of the work.

Working in a team requires careful preparation. It is usually helpful if the team elects a chairperson (this role can rotate around the group members) – it generally leads to more productive meetings. Each meeting should have an agenda. The chairperson has responsibility for ensuring that all items are addressed. Another group member should be responsible for taking notes of the decisions made and the division of work. At the end of every meeting all group members should agree and be clear about the tasks that they are to undertake. If the project is to be successful cooperation in planning, commitment to the group effort and adherence to agreed study protocols are essential. Unilateral decisions on the approach and methods by individuals regarding separate components of the project may undermine its integrity as a whole.

CONCLUSION

Investing time and effort at the preparatory stages of a project is usually immensely worthwhile. A systematic, thorough and thoughtful approach to the literature review and preliminary fieldwork is invaluable for ensuring the scientific validity of the research. Forethought in the overall planning of the project is vital for its successful completion. This includes devising a realistic time plan for the work, preparing applications for ethical approval early, and allowing sufficient time for all stages right through to the writing up and final presentation of the project. Smooth operation of the project will be greatly enhanced by setting up appropriate administrative procedures, such as meetings with collaborators and systematic organisation and filing.

2

Types of study:
design and approaches

This chapter provides an overview of the different types of study that are undertaken in pharmacy practice and related research, and the commonly employed study designs. As approaches to research in this field are often distinguished as quantitative or qualitative, a brief explanation of the purposes and features of the two approaches is also included. The selection of a suitable study design for a project depends principally on its overall aim. Specific objectives will determine the most appropriate approaches and methods.

In terms of their overall aims, most studies:

O describe or document current practices, events, behaviours or views in relation to pharmacy services or some aspect of the use of medicines

O assess current services or evaluate the effects of an intervention.

DESCRIPTIVE STUDIES

The aim of these studies is to describe or document phenomena, e.g.

O activities undertaken by pharmacists or other health professionals

O behaviour of consumers with regard to their medicines

O view or attitudes of individuals with regard to an aspect of their practice.

Descriptive studies are important when there is no systematic information. It is true that, for many of the activities that are undertaken in relation to pharmacy services or the use of medicines, we may believe that we have a good idea about what happens. Even if there is no systematic research, we may feel that, based on our own experience, that of our peers or anecdotal reports, we can estimate the frequency of different types of event in a health or pharmacy setting. We may believe that we have a good idea of the extent of certain health-related behaviours, the range of concerns of individuals with regard to different services, or how commonly particular views are held. However, if there is no systematic and accurate documentation of these phenomena, we cannot be sure about the true picture. If the sampling procedures are unscientific or unclear, we cannot draw inferences and generalise the information to other groups of people or settings. Also, we would not have adequate information to investigate any associations between the issue of interest and other factors (e.g. whether or not certain groups of patients are more likely to experience problems with their medicines, or whether there are any associations between the location of pharmacies and the demand for different services). Descriptive studies:

○   provide important data for informing people inside and outside the profession about pharmacy services and the use of medicines, and how and why these may vary

○   provide baseline information for investigating what is and is not good about services

○   enable the assessment of whether services are meeting health-care needs and identification of ways in which services should be improved

○   are an essential starting point for planning any changes to services or interventions.

Descriptive studies are often relatively straightforward in their design. However, these studies also require the careful selection of approaches, methods and measures if the data are to be valid and meaningful.

EVALUATION OF SERVICES

The aim of many studies is to evaluate either an aspect of current practice or a new service. The scope and range of services offered by pharmacists are developing fast. Many pharmacists are committed to extending and improving the services that they offer. They also recognise the need to assess which developments meet the needs of clients and are feasible in a practice setting.

An evaluation study will often focus on two areas. First, when a new service is introduced this will usually be with very specific objectives in mind (often related to improvements in some aspect of patient care). Thus, the evaluation will include an assessment of whether or not (and the extent to which) the new service has achieved its intended effect. Second, changes to service provision may also present problems, some of which may not be anticipated. When evaluating a service development, potential problems must also be identified. These may relate to its workability in different practice settings, its acceptability to health professionals, other staff or clients, logistical problems in its implementation, etc. Thus, the evaluation will assess the following:

○   The *effectiveness* of the intervention: does it achieve its objectives (e.g. in improving the service to patients)?

○   The *feasibility*: is the intervention workable for the professionals involved, and acceptable to clients? What problems arise in its implementation?

The design of studies to evaluate new services or to assess the impact of an intervention can be complex. A range of research approaches, methods and measures may be employed.

STUDY DESIGN

A wide range of terms can be used to describe the design of a study. Some of the most common design features and their application in pharmacy practice and related research are discussed below.

Many descriptive studies are *cross-sectional* in that data are collected from the population on one occasion only. Cross-sectional designs are probably the most common in health services research. Most questionnaire studies are cross-sectional, e.g. in a descriptive study investigating the activities or views of health professionals, patients or other participants, the researcher will often interview or survey the sample on a single occasion only. In addition, the information requested is commonly either *retrospective* (i.e. relating to what has happened in the past) or concerns the present time or situation. In some cases respondents are requested to maintain records of events, symptoms, etc. over a period of time (e.g. keep a diary). Thus, the study may be *prospective*, i.e. collecting data relating to the future.

Some studies are described as *exploratory*. These commonly employ qualitative methodology (see below) with the aim of investigating a topic from the perspective of different stakeholders and identifying the issues that are important to them. Sometimes they are also *hypothesis generating*, in that they provide clues about the important factors that may influence the behaviour of individuals, the success of a service, etc.

A *longitudinal study* follows up a sample of individuals over a period of time. Data will be collected from each individual on more than one occasion. These studies are sometimes called *cohort studies* (i.e. a group or cohort of individuals is followed for a given period), and may be descriptive in that a single population is followed up and their experiences described. Alternatively, the study may follow two or more cohorts to enable a comparison of their experiences over a period of time. An example would be a study that followed and compared cohorts of students from two or more different schools of pharmacy over a period of time.

Experimental studies are designed to test a hypothesis. Clinical trial design (in particular the *randomised controlled trial* or RCT) falls into this category. In health service and pharmacy practice research an experimental design can sometimes be used to assess the impact of a new service or intervention. However, in practice they are often not feasible. For example, to assess the impact of layout or other structural features in community pharmacies, it may not be possible to randomise (or impose upon) already established pharmacies. In an intervention study, ethical considerations may mean that patients should be offered a choice of services and may be aware of which they are receiving. In these cases an alternative study design, such as a *quasi-experimental design*, may be employed (see below).

An *intervention study* is designed to assess the impact of a change (i.e. a service development or intervention). The selection of an appropriate study design is essential if the research is to be of value. First, baseline data will be required. This will enable an assessment of whether or not the intervention resulted in any change (*before-and-after design*). Second, to be sure that any change was a direct result of the intervention and not some other factor(s), a control group is also needed (before-and-after design with a control group may constitute an *experimental* or *quasi-experimental design*).

For example, a *before-and-after design* may be employed to evaluate the impact of a drug information service on prescribing. Data relevant to the anticipated effects of the service are collected before the introduction of the service and again after its implementation. The difficulty that this design presents is that you cannot be sure whether or not any change was attributable to the service itself, rather than to other factors. To address this problem, a more robust design would include a control group, which should be similar in all respects to the group of individuals who are receiving the service (the intervention group), except that they do not experience the drug information service. If changes occurred in the intervention group, but not the control group, they could be attributed to the intervention. If individuals were randomised to either the control or intervention group, this would be an example of experimental design. If randomisation is not possible, individuals in the two groups could be *matched* (see Chapter 3), thus resulting in a *quasi-experimental design*.

The *evaluation* of services will often involve a range of objectives relating to patient care as well as implications for professionals, patients, health organisations and health policy. All these potential impacts should be taken into account in the design of the evaluation. In addition, service developments are implemented in natural settings (i.e. in the context of a wide variety of healthcare or pharmacy settings, situations and circumstances). To take all these 'real world' factors into account, a *holistic approach* to study design is desirable. This may entail a complex design, a combination of different methodological approaches and the measurement of a wide range of variables relating to aspects of the structures, processes and outcomes of the intervention.

Feasibility studies are often small-scale studies that aim to assess aspects of the efficacy or practicalities of an intervention. They are generally undertaken in a small number of selected settings and often focus on specific features of the service that would be deemed essential for its success (e.g. clinical efficacy or acceptability to health professionals or patients). If the feasibility study demonstrates that the service *can work* (albeit in a limited range of settings), it may then be reasonable to extend it to a wider range of situations. A broader evaluation of the service may then follow which asks '*does it work?*' when offered in a typical range of practice settings, under different circumstances and/or among various patient groups.

QUANTITATIVE AND QUALITATIVE APPROACHES

The approaches and methods of health service and pharmacy practice research are often distinguished as quantitative or qualitative.

Survey work, involving questionnaires or structured interviews, and studies in which numbers of events are counted, such as direct observation, records of prospective events or database analysis, is an example of quantitative research. Thus, quantitative methods are employed to investigate frequencies of events that may involve calculation of summary statistics, to establish the proportion of a population who hold certain views or have had particular experiences. That is, they are applied to research problems that require counting procedures to quantify phenomena of interest. They are also used to quantify relationships between variables (e.g. the use of statistical procedures to investigate associations between the variables in a database) or test a hypothesis (as in an experimental study).

The applications of quantitative studies contrast sharply with qualitative work, which is used to answer 'how?' and 'why?' questions. For example, we may want to investigate why people (health professionals or patients) behave in particular ways: what are their beliefs, concerns or priorities regarding their health, pharmacy services and use of medicines, and how do these affect what they do? To what extent can beliefs or behaviours be explained by their experiences or circumstances?

Qualitative studies are often exploratory, i.e. they attempt to identify possible explanations for particular phenomena. For this reason they are sometimes referred to as hypothesis generating. They are also commonly descriptive studies and they describe issues from the perspectives of respondents and in the context of their situations and circumstances. Qualitative methods are sometimes employed in evaluation studies, e.g. to establish what aspects of a new service are important to clients, or to gain an assessment of the value of the programme based on their priorities and concerns.

The most common qualitative approach in health services research is the qualitative interview. This is an unstructured interviewing technique that is flexible and responsive to the interviewee's agenda. It is challenging technique that requires skill on the part of the researcher (see Chapter 4).

Focus groups and participant observation are also usually employed as qualitative techniques.

Triangulation

Quantitative and qualitative approaches are seen as emerging from two distinct research paradigms. However, in health services research the value of combining quantitative and qualitative approaches to meet specific research aims and objectives is well recognised. Triangulation refers to the application of at least two different types of approach, method or data within a single research project. In health services research, triangulation is employed to:

○ provide different perspectives on a set of issues related to the study aims and objectives

○ obtain data on different issues and/or from a range of sources, which are relevant to the aims and objectives of the research

○ investigate, or demonstrate, the validity of data (by comparing data on the same variables that have been obtained in different ways).

CONCLUSION

Selection of the most suitable design, approach and method for a study is vital for meeting its aims and objectives. This chapter has provided an overview of the important principles in choosing a research design. As a result of their traditional science-based education, pharmacists are often more comfortable employing quantitative techniques. The science associated with pursuing qualitative methods is challenging for scientists unfamiliar with these approaches. However, qualitative methods are recognised as invaluable for the identification of needs, problems and possible solutions that may inform health policy. The strengths and weaknesses of different methods are discussed in greater detail in Chapter 4.

3

Selecting the sample and recruiting the participants

The principles of sampling and the application of procedures (probability and non-probability) in different types of pharmacy practice research are described in this chapter. The recruitment of participants is then discussed, in particular focusing on the problem of response rates, which is of importance in all studies.

SOURCES OF DATA

In much pharmacy practice and related research data are obtained from individuals. These may be pharmacists or other health professionals, pharmacy clients, members of the public, university students, etc. Documents are another source of data, e.g. information maintained on a database (such as prescription records), or documents relating to particular activities (such as records of drug information queries). Once the aims and objectives of the study have been determined, the population (i.e. the people who form the subject of study) or other potential data sources should be apparent.

POPULATIONS AND SAMPLES

The *population* are the people the study is about. As it is often impractical and unnecessary to gather data from everyone in a population (as in a census), a sample is commonly selected. The sampling procedure is of vital importance to the generalisability (or *external validity*) of the research. Provided that basic sampling principles are observed, the study will provide information that can be generalised or extrapolated to the whole study population.

The most important principle in selecting a sample is that it should be random. A random sample is also called a probability sample. This means that the probability of any member of the population being included in the sample can be calculated. Provided that a probability sampling procedure is followed, statistical procedures (which are also based on probabilities) can be applied. This enables a statement to be made about the likely accuracy of the information (i.e. estimates based on the sample) when it is generalised to the whole population.

SAMPLING PROCEDURES

A random sampling procedure is the ideal. A *simple random sample* is the most common and straightforward, but sometimes there are advantages to adopting more complex procedures, such as cluster sampling or stratified sampling, which can also be part of a random sampling process.

Non-random procedures (e.g. quota samples, snowball samples or convenience samples) present difficulties in ensuring representativeness, which leads to bias in the findings. Systematic differences between the sample and the population are called *sampling bias*.

For different types of study, e.g. experimental studies and qualitative research, there are further considerations and options.

A simple random sample

> A simple random sample is one into which every member of the population has an equal chance of being included.

To select a simple random sample, a list of all members of the population is required. This list is called the *sampling frame*. Everyone on the list is given a number, starting with 1. The size of the sample required must be decided (see below), sometimes as a sampling fraction (e.g. 1 in 10 sample). The sample is then selected using randomly generated numbers until the required sample size is reached.

If a sampling frame is available, selecting a simple random sample is a very straightforward procedure. Unless there are practical problems of collecting data from a simple random sample (e.g. interviewing individuals widely dispersed geographically), the procedure should be followed because it greatly enhances the value of the research.

The simple random sample also depends on the availability of a sampling frame. In many countries the names and addresses of registered pharmacies or local medical practitioners will be held by health organisations or professional bodies, and lists of students will be maintained by educational institutions. However, confidentiality and data protection may restrict access to the information by researchers. Comprehensive lists are also not available for all populations.

Addressing the difficulties of non-availability of a sampling frame can be time and resource consuming. You may need to construct your own sampling frame or develop an alternative strategy:

○ If information (names and addresses of individuals) required for sampling is not in the public domain (as is frequently the case in health services research), you may have to collaborate with health personnel (who have legitimate access to the information) to undertake the sampling and recruitment on your behalf.

○   For hospital pharmacists: a sampling frame could be constructed by contacting the hospitals of interest and obtaining information from each about the population of interest. The collective list could then form the sampling frame.

○   For pharmacy clients: a procedure sometimes adopted to obtain a random sample is to select perhaps every fourth, tenth and twentieth person who comes to the pharmacy (depending on the sample size needed). It is also important to select people at different times of the day, and perhaps on different days of the week, to ensure that the sample is representative of all clients.

○   Obtaining a population-based sample is generally difficult and expensive. Some government surveys use address files by post code to select participants.

The simple random sample is the most straightforward and effective probability sample. However, some useful modifications are stratified samples and cluster samples.

Stratified samples

A stratified sample is one in which the population is divided into subgroups (or strata) before selection. Stratification is particularly useful for making sure that small samples are representative. If the sample size is small, sampling error may lead to non-representation of small subgroups, e.g. a simple random sample of pharmacists, if very small, may not include individuals from minority groups. By dividing the sample into categories (or strata) before you undertake random selection, you can ensure that all groups are represented. A simple random sampling procedure is then adopted for all strata. The sample is called a *stratified random sample*.

If the sample frame is stratified, proportionate numbers of individuals in each subgroup can be selected (e.g. 10%). For example, in a study of pharmacy students, you may wish to ensure that individuals from different years of study are similarly represented. In other studies it may be appropriate to sample disproportionately, e.g. in research among pharmacists with different levels of experience or specialisation, the population may include very small numbers in some specialities. To ensure a minimum number from all groups, you may need to select a higher proportion from some strata than others.

Cluster samples

A cluster sample is one in which the sample is drawn from a limited number of study sites (i.e. clustered in particular locations). This is useful for populations spread over a wide geographical area. The area is divided up into locations and data collection concentrated in a random sample of these locations. Restricting the data collection to a smaller number of study sites may mean that you can include more individuals from each of these sites (i.e. data collection will be more efficient). A cluster sample is often drawn in several stages, e.g. to study an aspect of pharmacy services across the country you may decide to focus your study on a number of geographical locations. You may begin by randomly selecting a small number of regions of the country and then smaller localities within each of these regions. This may make the study more manageable than selecting a simple random sample of pharmacies from a national sampling frame.

Stratification is sometimes combined with cluster sampling, e.g. if data collection is going to be concentrated in a small number of geographical areas, you may wish to stratify each location in terms of whether urban or rural, or on the basis of socioeconomic variables. This would ensure that the areas selected were representative in terms of these characteristics.

Non-probability sampling procedures

Sometimes it is not possible to select a truly random sample. This occurs if no sampling frame can be found or constructed. Under these circumstances, a non-random sampling procedure may be considered. The researcher then has to find the best possible procedure to obtain a sample that is as representative as possible of the population. Even though the procedure is not random, the researcher may ensure that it includes representative numbers of men and women, people living in different areas or people of different educational levels, or other features deemed important to the objectives of the study.

Non-random samples are not ideal. Ensuring that they are representative can be problematic: however hard you try, the sampling will be open to some bias. When reporting the study findings possible bias in the sampling, and its implications, must be addressed. If a non-random sampling procedure is followed, the sample cannot be described as a probability sample. The application of probability statistics may be inappropriate. Great care must be taken before suggesting the wider applicability of the study findings. Examples of non-probability samples include quota samples, membership lists of voluntary organisations, snowball samples and convenience samples.

Quota samples have commonly been used in market research. Quota samples in some respects may be representative of the population under study. They include specific numbers of individuals from different age groups, male and female respondents, and individuals from different socio-economic groups. Thus, the researcher can claim that the sample included people with different personal characteristics, and may feel that they can draw some inferences about the wider population on the basis of the selection procedure, but, because the participants were not randomly selected, the sampling procedure is open to sampling bias which will have implications for the study findings.

Snowball sampling is a technique that has been used to recruit members of an otherwise inaccessible and usually small population. The principle is that one member of a population is identified and recruited and further participants are contacted through the network of this individual. This is clearly open to serious bias, but the technique may be justified in situations when there is no other way of accessing a population to investigate important healthcare issues.

Convenience samples are those in which the researcher selects individuals who are most accessible and willing to take part. Even though individuals from varied backgrounds may be included, they cannot be assumed to be representative of the study population. However, convenience samples are useful in preliminary fieldwork and pilot studies. In these cases generalisability is less important because the goal of the researcher is often to assess the feasibility of the methodology. Otherwise convenience samples should be used only if there is no way of obtaining a more representative sample.

Membership lists of voluntary organisations can sometimes be used as a sampling frame. Although they may include a large number of individuals and provide the scope for a large sample, it must be remembered that these members will be a self-selecting group. They would be expected to share some common background and/or interests, e.g. members of a self-help group may include disproportionate numbers of individuals who have experienced greater problems in the management of their condition and, on this basis, will be unrepresentative of the total population who share their diagnosis.

A *self-selecting sample* is one in which people choose to take part. Self-selecting samples are likely to include people with a special interest in the topic area and who are therefore unrepresentative of the population as a whole.

An element of self-selection colours many sampling procedures. Even when a random sampling procedure is followed, participants who agree to take part will be self-selecting. This is referred to as *response bias* (see below) and it presents similar difficulties with regard to representativeness as sampling bias.

SAMPLING IN EXPERIMENTAL OR INTERVENTION STUDIES

When sampling for experimental or intervention studies, many of the principles of random selection still apply. However, as a result of the design of the study, there are additional considerations.

The design of an experimental study will generally include both an intervention and a control group. If possible, individuals should be randomly assigned to one or other of these groups, as in a clinical trial. However, in health services research this is not always possible, e.g. in many cases people must be allowed to choose between service options or the type of therapy that they want. They cannot just be assigned to receive a particular type of care irrespective of their preferences. To address this difficulty a quasi-experimental design may be used in which random allocation is replaced by matching in an attempt to achieve equivalence between the two groups. *Matching* involves identification of the important characteristics of the individuals or setting that are believed to be associated with study outcomes. Then, for each participant in the intervention group, an individual displaying similar characteristics is identified and recruited to the control group. Thus, participants in the intervention and control groups are matched on the variables of importance.

Matching is not as good as random allocation because there may be factors that distinguish individuals in the intervention group from the control group which have not been identified or cannot be matched for. However, it is a common technique and may be the best option when random allocation to intervention and control groups is not possible.

SAMPLING FOR EVALUATION STUDIES THAT DO NOT EMPLOY AN EXPERIMENTAL DESIGN

In the evaluation of many health and pharmacy service developments, a range of approaches can be employed. As many health service interventions have implications for health authorities, health professionals, patients and others, representatives of all these groups may be included in the evaluation. For example, the success of the new service may be measured in terms of its pre-specified objectives, and/or the anticipated and unanticipated outcomes, benefits, costs, etc. from the perspectives of different stakeholders. When a holistic approach is taken a range of sampling strategies may be required. These may depend on the availability of suitable sampling frames for each population group. Thus, within a study, different approaches may be required for the selection of patients and health professionals, or for health professionals in primary and secondary care. However, in all cases, the principles of probability sampling should be followed if possible.

SAMPLING OF DOCUMENTS FOR ANALYSIS

For many research studies the data-sets are derived from sources other than individuals. The information required to meet the study objectives may be available within an existing data-set (e.g. prescribing information maintained by health organisations or hospital pharmacies). The project may focus on records maintained by practitioners (e.g. records of medication errors or requests for drug information) or data maintained by educational institutions (e.g. students and their performance). The study may be an analysis of other written documents (e.g. drug policy guidelines, medicines information available to consumers). When relying on existing data-sets as a source of data, decisions have to be made about their completeness and reliability and also whether or not they are sufficiently comprehensive to meet the study objectives.

Again, in the selection of material, similar principles should be followed. For example, if investigating prescribing patterns, the data-set should be representative of prescribers with different characteristics, in different geographical areas or healthcare settings, etc. In examining medicines information available to consumers, the sampling of documents must take into account the full range of sources relevant to the study objectives.

SAMPLING FOR QUALITATIVE STUDIES

Sampling in qualitative studies is not necessarily probability based. The aims and objectives of qualitative research are generally effectively met by detailed work with small samples. The high level of sampling error expected with small samples means that other procedures are often more appropriate. Random sampling may be appropriate if the population is very small (and consequently the sampling fraction is large). In some studies, random sampling after stratification may be the best approach.

Purposive samples

In qualitative research *purposive sampling* is commonly adopted. Purposive sampling is a non-random procedure. Its scientific validity rests on the basis that it is theoretically informed, i.e. the researcher has preconceived ideas about the required characteristics of the sample. These are based on the aims and objectives of the study along with established theories about relevant explanatory variables identified in earlier research. On this basis, the researcher purposively identifies and selects those individuals who would be expected to be the most informative in meeting the study objectives, e.g. targeted individuals may be those who have had particular experiences or high- or low-level involvement with a particular programme, are influential in decision-making about service development, or have other specified important characteristics pertinent to the study. Although small and non-random, a purposive sample is not a convenience sample. The sampling strategy in terms of the theoretical rationale and the selection procedure must be clearly described and convincingly justified by the researcher.

Sampling for focus groups

Focus group research is generally viewed as a qualitative procedure. In some instances random selection of groups or individual participants will be possible and the most appropriate means of meeting study objectives. However, the study may aim to explore in detail the perspectives of individuals who share particular experiences, interests and backgrounds; in these cases a purposive sampling procedure may be more suitable. In the selection of samples for focus groups a number of additional issues must be considered.

Should you include established groups or convene them for the purposes of the study?

If suitable existing groups can be identified this can reduce the administrative burden on the researcher. Contacting such groups is generally less onerous than convening your own. It often requires communication with only one group member rather than all. In established groups the members will usually know each other. They are, of course, self-selecting and would be expected to share some background characteristics and interests. This may provide the researcher with an opportunity to explore in detail issues with a group who are in a familiar environment and possibly relaxed in each other's company. This may be advantageous to the depth of discussion. As with all groups the discussion will be coloured by established group dynamics and relationships.

By convening the groups yourself (i.e. selecting each individual) you are able to ensure some degree of representativeness in the sample which may be important. Also, you can often retain control over the number of participants and the suitability of the setting for a group discussion more easily. Depending on the recruitment procedures and setting, the individual participants may or may not know each other. The discussion will still be influenced by group dynamics, inevitably including both more dominant and quieter participants (see Chapter 4).

How many groups?

The number of groups depends on the purpose of the study. Focus groups are sometimes used in the early stages of a research project to identify relevant issues that will then be addressed in more detail in a larger study; one or two groups may be sufficient for this. In other studies the minimum number of groups may be determined by the need to include a range of population groups.

How many participants in each group?

Group size is known to be an important influence on the effective functioning of a group. Large groups may hinder the development of an in-depth discussion but a wider range of issues may be raised. Optimum group size is generally considered to be five to seven participants. As group size increases, the number of quiet or non-contributing members tends to rise.

SAMPLE SIZE

Quantitative studies

The statistical approach to determining the required sample size in quantitative studies is to perform a power calculation. In experimental studies this is based on estimations of the differences on important variables between groups. For a given sample size and level of statistical significance, it provides a measure of the likelihood that a difference between groups will be detected.

In survey research the sample size required is determined by the degree of accuracy desired when the estimate based on the sample is applied to the wider population. In general the larger the sample size the more accurate the estimates (and the narrower the confidence intervals) will be when extrapolated to the wider population. If subgroup analyses (see Chapter 5) are to be performed, it is also important to ensure that there will be sufficient numbers of cases in each subgroup. In deciding the sample size the anticipated response rate is also a determining factor.

Power calculations and determination of an appropriate sample size can be complicated, depending on the design of the study and the aims of the research. Practical considerations, in particular time and resource constraints, also have to be taken into account. In some cases, reference to appropriate texts and/or advice from a statistician will be required.

It is important to remember that increasing the sample size will not address the problem of sampling bias (non-representativeness resulting from non-random sampling procedures), although sampling error (random error that results from a small sampling fraction) will be reduced. Also, an increase in the sample size will not compensate for non-representativeness that results from poor response rates (i.e. response bias).

Qualitative studies

There are no hard-and-fast rules about the determination of the appropriate sample size for qualitative research, and power calculations are generally not appropriate.

In qualitative research sample sizes are generally small to allow for the detailed work in the data processing and analysis. In exploratory studies that aim to identify the relevant issues in relation to a topic of interest, sampling and data collection continue until no new issues emerge. This is sometimes referred to as *saturation sampling*. If a purposive procedure and the principles of qualitative enquiry are followed, the study objectives will often be effectively met with a small sample.

Sample size issues for focus groups, in terms of numbers of groups and participants are discussed above.

RECRUITING THE PARTICIPANTS

Once the sample has been selected the next task is the recruitment of the participants. Eligibility criteria, both inclusion and exclusion, should be clear.

For a postal survey a covering letter and reply-paid envelope is generally included with the self-completion questionnaire. It is usual to send out two reminders at appropriate time intervals (e.g. 3 weeks apart).

Questionnaires should be coded so that non-responders can be identified for repeat mailings and/or, in the case of persistent non-response, for follow-up. This is important. Omitting these codes (to provide anonymity) has not been shown to lead to an increase in response rates. In addition, inability to assess the implications of non-response for the study findings is a shortcoming that can seriously affect the value of the research. Knowledge of the respondents also allows the researcher to acknowledge receipt and thank respondents for their participation. The covering letter should assure potential respondents that confidentiality will be maintained and that no one will be identifiable in the results of the study. Although the covering letter should be brief and to the point, it should also inform potential participants of the purposes (or aims and objectives) of the research, how and why they have been selected, by whom the research is being funded and conducted, what it will involve for them, and who to contact for further information. It is also usual to include details relating to approval by the relevant ethics committees.

Potential participants may be invited to an interview by you in person as the researcher, by a third party or by post. If researchers undertake this themselves, they can be sure that recruitment procedures are followed and that details of non-response or declines are noted. However, for reasons of confidentiality of information this sometimes has to be done by a health professional with legitimate access to records. Recruitment of interviewees may also be done by mail or telephone. When invitations to participate are forwarded by mail (often preferable for patients or members of the public), it is usual to include a covering letter (as above), an information leaflet about the study (see Chapter 1), a reply slip and reply-paid envelope, and sometimes a consent form. Telephone recruitment is sometimes used for health professionals. Information about the study can be forwarded before the telephone call. The provision of information in advance gives people an opportunity to consider their involvement before the telephone call and decide whether they are willing to make arrangements for an interview there and then. Similar procedures may be employed for the recruitment of focus group participants. Information leaflets should be available for all participants.

RESPONSE RATES AND NON-RESPONDERS

One of the biggest problems for researchers is non-response. Any response rate below 100% opens up the study to response bias. Many researchers have demonstrated that non-responders may differ from responders in important ways and that this results in bias in the study findings. Maximising response rates and addressing non-responses must be seen as an important part of any project.

Response rates of, or near, 100% are rare. They are generally achieved only in 'captive' populations when the researcher is on site, or when potential participants feel obliged to take part (which suggests an ethical problem).

Response rates vary dramatically. When high response rates are not achieved (whatever strategy was used in the sample selection), the sample must be viewed as self-selecting (i.e. of doubtful representativeness regarding the population). This potentially undermines the scientific validity of the work, e.g. it is likely that, in any study, people with a particular interest in the research area would be more likely to respond, and in this they will differ from non-responders.

For researchers there are two important issues. The importance of these cannot be underestimated. They will require time and effort. They are:

○   maximising the response rate, to reduce the level of response bias

○   assessing the impact of the response bias on the study findings.

Maximising response rates

Steps to achieve as high a response rate as possible must be a priority. Possible reasons why people may be reluctant should be identified in advance and these should be addressed in the recruitment procedures. For example:

○   Potential participants may show a lack of interest in the study area. The purposes of the work, drawing out its ultimate value, should be emphasised.

○   Potential participants may be unclear about what the study will involve and/or how the results might be used. Make sure that these issues are explained in the initial contact (covering letter, information leaflet or telephone conversation). Be prepared to answer all questions to allay any suspicions. Sources of funding, who is conducting the work and the motives for undertaking it should be stated.

○ Potential participants may believe that they will have little to contribute. Explain the sampling procedures and the need for representativeness if the results are to be valid. Stress that all contributions are equally important. It should be clear that you have no prior expectations.

○ Potential participants may be very busy and perceive that the study may interfere with normal working. Researchers should ensure that questionnaires/interviews are as concise as possible. The layout should be attractive and easy to follow; realistic estimates of the anticipated time involved should be given. Payment in lieu of time (and/or other expenses) could be considered. At the outset you should consider if what you are asking participants to do is reasonable. Methods that require minimal input or inconvenience on the part of the participant should be devised.

○ Potential participants may be concerned about confidentiality. In the covering letter and information leaflet assurances should be given that data will be treated confidentially, that no one will be identifiable in the results, and that the study will have met accepted ethical standards.

These and other steps taken to maximise response rates should be described when writing up the project.

Assessing the impact of the response bias on the study findings

Non-responders should be followed up to establish how they differ from responders. Some information on non-responders may be apparent from the sampling frame. However, this is generally restricted to a few personal or workplace character-istics, e.g. gender, geographical location, whether pharma-cists are from independent, small or large pharmacies, whether medical practitioners are in single-handed or mul-tiple practices. This information, although worth reporting, may not be of major importance for the research findings. Information on variables important to the research may be established only by direct communication (e.g. by telephone) with a sample (preferably random) of non-responders. Only limited information can generally be obtained at this time, so this investigation should focus on a few key variables that are important to the study objectives. These data can then be taken into account in the analysis and interpretation of the findings.

An alternative approach that has sometimes been used in survey research is to compare the data obtained from early and late responders, i.e. received in response to the first and final mailings. The basis of this approach is that variation between early and late responders may reflect differences between responders and non-responders, i.e. non-responders would be expected to be more similar to late responders. If this analysis is to be conducted the time of receipt of each questionnaire must be noted.

CONCLUSION

Although a probability sample is the ideal, the simple random sample being the most straightforward procedure, this approach is not always possible. In these cases careful thought must be given to establish the best alternative. What is of great importance is that you are aware of the compromises of the procedures that you have employed and that you critically consider the implications for the study findings.

Difficulties can also arise in recruitment of participants, such that even if an optimal sampling procedure has been followed the representativeness of the sample is in doubt. You may have limited control over your recruitment (e.g. as a result of ethical constraints and access to information for sampling). Non-response, too, can jeopardise the scientific validity of a study. Opportunities for following up non-responders to assess potential response bias may be limited. However, every effort must be made to address these problems and to assess their possible impact on your results. In this regard you should be prepared to describe and justify your approaches and methods and demonstrate your awareness of their potential effects.

4

Methods of data collection and research instruments

This chapter provides an overview of different ways of collecting data and their strengths and weaknesses when applied to pharmacy and related settings. The actual data required for a study are determined by its objectives. The objectives also indicate whether a quantitative or qualitative approach is appropriate.

In terms of study methods, sometimes there will different ways of collecting the data. For example, survey data could be gathered by self-completion questionnaire or in interviews. The best method may then depend on factors such as the required sample size, the geographical spread of the population or sample, the likely response rates from each approach, etc. Data relating to events could be collected by the study participants, who may be asked to keep a diary or maintain records of events. Data could also be collected by the researcher, e.g. by direct observation in the practice setting or the analysis of retrospective records if these exist. Again, each of these approaches has its advantages and disadvantages. Asking participants to maintain diaries can be time-consuming for them and the researcher may have a problem verifying the reliability and completeness of information. Observation by a researcher is expensive and may limit the number of sites that can be included in the sample. Analysis of records assumes that all relevant data are available, but frequently key variables may not be included in the data-set.

Issues of reliability and validity arise in all studies.

Reliability

> Reliability refers to the extent to which procedures, measures and data are reproducible or internally consistent.

Problems of reliability may arise in relation to repeated measures on a piece of diagnostic equipment, uniformity between researchers in the collection of data, adherence of interviewers to an interview schedule, completeness in maintaining records of non-responders, care and attentiveness when observing events, consistency of responses to questions in a questionnaire, etc. In the development of research instruments and data collection procedures, potential problems with regard to the reliability of data must be identified and addressed.

Validity

> Validity refers to the extent to which the measures (e.g. questions in an interview, records maintained by an observer) actually measure what they are designed to measure.

All methods present their own concerns with regard to the validity of data and are discussed later in this chapter. However, some common examples are that, when people are being observed, they may modify their behaviour in a systematic way so that the data are not an accurate reflection of a true situation or, in a questionnaire, respondents may tend to underestimate on some variables (e.g. their smoking habits) and overestimate on others. Potential problems in the validity of data must also be identified and addressed. External validity, or generalisability, is important in sampling strategies, recruitment procedures and response rates (see Chapter 3). Issues of reliability and validity are also important in the data processing and analysis (see Chapter 5).

The following are common methods of data collection in pharmacy practice research.

Quantitative studies

○   Questionnaires

○   Interviews (structured or semi-structured)

○   Non-participant observation

○   Prospective recording of activities or events

○   Retrospective analysis of data-sets maintained for other purposes.

Qualitative studies

○   Interviews (semi-structured or unstructured)

○   Focus groups (group interviews)

○   Observation (participant and non-participant).

Each of these methods is discussed in terms of its application or use in research, its principal strengths and weaknesses (including any particular difficulties that it presents), the development of instruments, issues of reliability and validity, and other possible ways of collecting similar data.

QUESTIONNAIRES

Survey research using questionnaires is the most commonly adopted method in pharmacy practice research. In many studies this will be the sole approach; in others, a questionnaire may be just one component. Frequently questionnaires are for self-completion by the respondent, although they may also be completed by researchers in interviews.

Questionnaires can be very useful for collecting information from large samples relatively cheaply, and generally in a reasonably short time. Costs include administration, postage (for repeated mailings and return of questionnaires), and perhaps telephone follow-up of non-responders. The time required can easily be underestimated. Devoting sufficient time to developing and validating the instrument is vital if the data are to be useful. Obtaining a sampling frame is not always straightforward. It is usual to send two reminders, (e.g. 3 weeks apart) and additional time will be absorbed in waiting for the return of completed questionnaires. Time should be dedicated to the follow-up of non-responders. Although some data processing (e.g. coding or setting up of the database) can be undertaken when waiting for responses, the analysis is more efficiently started only when all data have been received.

A major difficulty of survey research is achieving a good response rate. Low response rates (which are not uncommon) can jeopardise the value of the research. Careful consideration should be given to maximising the response rate (see Chapter 3). Points relevant to the instrument itself are raised below. Some assessment of response bias should also be attempted (see Chapter 3).

Although questionnaires are seen as an efficient method of data collection from large numbers of individuals, this does depend on the data required. They are considered good for factual data, but this assumes that people are able to provide the relevant information, e.g. people may have difficulty recalling the last time they visited a pharmacy, how long they have been taking a particular medicine, or the names of medicines they are currently using. People may be unwilling to provide some information (e.g. relating to personal or business issues) or they may not know the answers to some questions. They may, in an effort to be helpful, make unsubstantiated guesses, or their responses may be influenced by their perceptions of the purposes of the questionnaire and the researchers' expectations. These potential problems may undermine the reliability and the validity of the data.

Instrument development

The questionnaire is referred to as the *research instrument*. Constructing the questionnaire is an important part of a research project. It is worth investing time and effort at this stage. If the questionnaire is poor, this will be reflected in the data obtained. Once the questionnaire has been mailed there is no opportunity to take any remedial action to review or revise question structures, add items or correct errors, i.e. 'garbage in, garbage out'. Conversely, if the instrument has been rigorously prepared, issues of validity and reliability have been fully considered and attention has been paid to the presentation, covering letter, etc., then much of the complex work has been done. The data processing will be straightforward and the analysis will not be hampered by concerns over the quality of the data.

The first issue to consider when developing the questionnaire is the content. What information is needed to meet the study objectives? Identification and coverage of all relevant issues are referred to as the content validity. Content validity must be achieved from the perspective of the population under study. It is not safe, generally, to rely on a list generated by an individual group of researchers. There would usually be issues which they had perhaps thought not pertinent to particular settings, and the relative importance of related issues to the study population may be unclear. Thus, an important stage of construction of the questionnaire is preliminary fieldwork to ensure content validity of the instrument. This often takes the form of a small number of interviews with key individuals (often representatives of the study population) supported by a review of the literature. This process enables the identification of all issues relevant to the aims of the study, and assures the content validity.

Once all the relevant issues have been identified, questions have to be devised before being incorporated into the questionnaire. Again great care must be paid to the construction of the questions. The following are issues that must be considered for each question.

Questions may be closed or open

Closed questions include a 'stem' followed by a limited range of responses. Ensuring that the responses include all the likely answers is also an issue of *content validity* that should be addressed in the preliminary fieldwork or pilot work. The response options should be discrete and mutually exclusive, unless the question is intended to be multiple response (see below). Closed questions are often preferred in self-completion questionnaires. If well constructed they are quicker and easier for respondents to answer; they generally lead to fewer *missing data*; and they are easier for the researcher to code and incorporate into quantitative analyses.

Open questions provide an opportunity for freedom of expression in answering. These questions are more difficult to code because, in response to any question, everyone may say something different. This leaves the researcher with the difficult task of interpreting the data and categorising the responses. Also, in a questionnaire, answers are generally brief and there is no scope (as in an interview) for obtaining clarification or further details relating to a response to an open question.

Open questions are commonly included at the end of a questionnaire to allow respondents the opportunity to add any issues that they feel are important and have not been covered by the instrument. This can be a useful check on the content validity of the instrument.

Questions may use objective, subjective or relative quantifiers

Many questionnaires require respondents to estimate the frequency of events or the importance of particular issues.

In estimating the frequency of events respondents may be asked to make an objective assessment (e.g. daily, at least once a week, etc.) or a subjective assessment (e.g. rarely, fairly frequently, often, etc.). Objective assessments (assuming these are reasonably accurate) enable the researcher to provide summary information about the actual frequency of events. Subjective assessments provide a picture of the perceptions of respondents of the frequencies compared with what they may believe to be the norm or an ideal. It is widely acknowledged that what is frequent for one person may not be for another. In constructing the questions, the researcher must ask him- or herself whether an objective or a subjective assessment is required.

Multiple response questions

Multiple response questions (closed questions in which respondents can select more than one response) are generally less straightforward when it comes to coding and analysis. It is important that it is clear to respondents how the question should be answered. Decisions have to be made in advance about how many responses will be allowed, whether they should be ranked in order of importance, etc. This will have implications for coding of data and analysis. If there is a lack of clarity in the directions, some respondents may treat the question as single response and others as a multiple response; this will require the researcher to make decisions about the respondents' true positions, which will threaten the validity of the data.

Questions that can be problematic

During preparation and pilot work the questionnaire should be carefully screened for potentially problematic questions. These include the following:

○   Questions in which respondents may have a problem in providing the requested information, i.e. when they do not know the answer, e.g. a pharmacist may not know whether a local surgery has specific policies relating to aspects of prescribing or patient care.

○   Questions requesting sensitive information, e.g. personal or business details that people are not happy to disclose.

○   Questions that are ambiguous and therefore likely to produce spurious, unreliable or missing data.

○   Double-barrelled questions (e.g. 'Are your colleagues on the ward friendly and helpful?') to which the researcher assumes a single answer can be given.

○   Questions that include a negative. These are more likely to be misread and should be kept to a minimum.

Asking respondents to express their views and assessing attitudes

Developing a questionnaire to assess attitudes is a complex task. Such questionnaires generally rely on items that ask respondents to express their views on a series of statements, which are assumed to represent the beliefs and values that underpin an individual's attitude. It is difficult to demonstrate objectively that the items accurately reflect the relevant components in terms of the beliefs, experiences and values (i.e. display content and construct validity). In addition, attention has to be paid to the capture and representation of the depth and breadth of feelings in relation to all these components. Many questionnaires in health service and pharmacy practice research, which claim to assess attitudes, merely request an individual's views on selected aspects of a topic. As such they are better described as a survey of views or opinions. If a true attitudinal measure is required it may be best to find an established and validated tool from the literature rather than attempt, in a limited period, to develop one of your own. If you are to embark on this, rigorous fieldwork will be required. Attention must be paid to the content and construct validity (i.e. all the relevant domains and issues identified and items accurately reflecting these), that statements represent different strengths of feeling in relation to different issues, to the balance of positive and negative items, etc. As in any questionnaire, all items must be reviewed to avoid potential problems arising from question structure or interpretation. Likert scales (strongly agree, agree, neither agree nor disagree, disagree, strongly disagree) are commonly used for responses to items in these questionnaires. As a Likert scale is not a true linear scale, care is required in the data analysis (see Chapter 5).

Reliability and validity in questionnaires

A number of issues about the reliability and validity of questionnaires have already been raised. However, in the case of questionnaires, reliability refers to the extent to which the questions lead to reproducible responses that are internally consistent. Factors that can lead to unreliability relate to question construction, e.g. those that are ambiguous or difficult for respondents to answer. Validity refers to the extent to which the questions provide a true measure of what they are designed to measure, e.g. in response to a question on smoking, smokers may consistently under-report; regarding their compliance with a medication regimen, they may tend to overestimate. Thus, the questions are of doubtful validity, even though they may be reliable in the sense that repeated questioning would provide the same results.

Different types of validity have been distinguished:

○ The first to be addressed in questionnaires is usually *face validity*, i.e. prima facie (without further investigation) would the question be expected to produce accurate information? Face-validity checks aim to uncover fairly obvious problems such as ambiguous questions or those that may be expected to lead to inaccurate responses. A check on face validity can be carried out by a request for a review of the instrument by experienced researchers and representatives of the study population.

O   *Criterion validity* refers to whether or not questions correlate with other measures of the same variable, e.g. it may be possible to check the validity of questions by comparison with data from other sources.

O   *Construct validity* is concerned with the extent to which questions accurately represent a concept or construct. For example, questions to establish the socioeconomic status of a respondent generally focus on occupation (sometimes education, home ownership, income, etc. are also used). These questions are assumed to be a valid indicator of what people term 'social class'.

O   *Content validity* (the extent to which data gathered cover all the issues relevant to the study objectives), in relation to questionnaire construction, has been discussed above.

General points about questionnaire structure and layout

The questionnaire should be headed with the title of the project together with a reminder of its principal aims. The presentation and layout should be clear and easy to follow. Respondents should not have to waste time working out which questions lead on from which, and where to move on to should a question be 'not applicable'.

Unlike an interview, it is assumed that respondents may look through the entire questionnaire before responding. Therefore, the order of questions is in some ways less important. However, some attention should be paid to this. The question order should be logical, so that the overall questionnaire structure is easily discernible. It is common to place questions relating to personal or professional information (age, sex, working situation, etc.) at the end of the instrument. Towards the end of the questionnaire it is also common to provide an opportunity for respondents to add any further comments that they believe are relevant.

A code (to identify the respondent) should be included at either the top or bottom of the questionnaire. This enables a follow-up of the non-responders, which is important for the study findings. There is no evidence that omission of an identifier (to confer anonymity) improves response rates. Names and addresses should not appear.

Other ways of collecting similar data

Many questionnaires that are designed for self-completion can also be used in an interview. In general, interviews are preferable for less structured instruments, which often comprise a higher proportion of open questions. Interviews provide an opportunity to follow up any ambiguous or interesting responses. They also enable some flexibility on the part of the interviewer in responding to, and exploring further, issues raised by the respondent that are deemed relevant to the study objectives. However, interviews are more labour intensive and a large sample size may have to be compromised if they are used as an alternative to self-completion questionnaires. Some data collected in a questionnaire could also be gathered through direct observation by a researcher. This has the advantage of providing data on actual events rather than a respondent's reports of these events. Again, because these studies are labour intensive a large sample may not be feasible.

INTERVIEWS

Research interviews are used to gather information from individuals, in particular when considered responses are required, and the researcher wishes to have the opportunity to explore the contexts, rationale and details of the interviewees' responses. Interviews are often used to explore issues from the perspective of the respondents in the light of their priorities, perceptions and experiences. They are employed in both quantitative and qualitative studies and in those that bridge the two.

Research interviews are commonly distinguished as *structured*, *semi-structured* or *unstructured* (*in-depth*). In general, a structured interview follows a structured questionnaire that differs from a self-completion questionnaire principally in that it is likely to include more open questions. It may also include instructions to the interviewer to clarify responses to ensure that data are comprehensive and comprehensible. Semi-structured interviews follow an *interview schedule*, which comprises mainly open questions. Thus, semi-structured interviews enable a more detailed exploration of issues raised by the respondent. This is probably the most common interview approach. The instrument is commonly called the interview schedule. 'Unstructured' interviews follow an *interview guide* that provides only a framework for the interview. The actual content of the interview, in terms of the issues discussed, is determined by the respondent's experiences, views, perceptions, etc. It is up to interviewers to use their skills to ensure that the interviews fully explore these perspectives rather than being influenced by their own agenda or preconceptions. However, some closed questions may be included to clarify the respondent's views on particular issues. Thus, the purpose of an unstructured interview is to explore issues from the perspective of the respondent. Patients' perspectives are increasingly seen as important in informing the future of healthcare. Interviews provide an opportunity to contribute to this research and policy agenda.

Developing the interview schedule and interviewing skills

The interview schedule, as a questionnaire, comprises a series of questions. The instruments differ in that, in an interview, a high proportion of the questions is open. Many probing questions are also often used, e.g. an open question may ask respondents what issues are important to them in relation to a topic. Once the respondent has outlined their views and thoughts on this, the interviewer may move on to probing questions to gather more detail on these views and associated experiences, e.g.

> Would you say more about . . .?
> What do you think are the reasons for . . .?

Question order matters. Open questions should always come before closed questions on the same issue. If the interviewer begins with questions on specific points, the respondent's thoughts may be channelled to these points to the exclusion of a more wide-ranging exposition of the issues from the respondent's point of view, i.e. the interviewer runs the risk of directing the interview down a particular path. Only when the interviewer believes that the respondent has no more to add in relation to any question should they request comments on specific points that they believe could be important.

Thus, typically the interview schedule will start with an open question requesting a respondent's views or experiences on a particular issue. Subsequent questioning will depend on the response to this open question, e.g. in probing questions the interviewer may request more description of actual events, reasons why particular views are held, their perspectives on how and why any problems arose, how these were or could be addressed, etc., depending on the objectives of the research. In some cases one or more closed questions may then follow. This will ensure that some comparable data on key issues are obtained from each respondent. The researcher can also check that they have correctly understood the respondent's viewpoint.

Semi-structured and unstructured interviews require particular skill on the part of the researcher. Unlike a questionnaire for which, once the instrument is devised, the role of the researcher in data collection is minimal, there is great skill in conducting an interview, applying the interview schedule and ensuring that relevant principles of qualitative enquiry are followed. The following are some general principles that must be observed by the interviewer.

Avoid leading questions

These are questions to which it is clear what answer is expected. Respondents are more likely to provide the expected response. Probing questions, to obtain additional detail on issues raised by the respondent, may or may not be needed. However, it can be very helpful to provide a list of non-leading follow-up questions in the interview schedule for the interviewer to use as needed.

Pace the interview

Semi-structured and unstructured interviews also require considered responses from the respondent. Thus, it is important that the pace of the interview allows for this. Silences in the interview are often necessary thinking time. Rushing in with further questions risks losing valuable information from the respondent. It can also result in poor questioning (such as use of leading questions); the interviewer needs thinking time too, to construct their questions.

Avoid interrupting the respondent

The goal of an interview is to obtain accurate information on the respondent's perspectives, priorities or concerns relating to an issue. Interrupting respondents may suggest to them that what they have to say is not important. It may interfere with their thought processes, resulting in the loss of relevant data, and may also make them more hesitant to express their views subsequently in the interview.

Make sure you listen, identify all the relevant issues raised by the respondent and follow them up

Listening is vital for the success of the interview. When responding to an open question a respondent may raise a number of relevant issues. However, unless prompted by the interviewer, he or she may not provide detail on all of them. It is important that the interviewer registers all of them and comes back to each in turn for further elucidation before leaving the question.

Location of interview and personal interaction

For a successful interview, the interviewer and the respondent should be comfortable and settled. For sensitive topics it is helpful if external interruptions are kept to a minimum. That you are paying attention to responses, interested in their perspectives and sympathetic to their concerns should be apparent from your body language.

So that the interviewer knows which questions are to be asked of all respondents, and which are to be used as needed to follow up responses, different typefaces in the interview schedule may be helpful, e.g. the following scheme could be used:

O   'starter' open questions to be asked of all respondents could be printed in bold type

O   prompts or probing questions to be used as needed could be in normal print

O   instructions to interviewers could be written in italics.

Conduct of an interview: developing your interviewing skills

Interviews (except structured interviews) are generally audio-recorded (with the permission of the respondent). Audio-recording, and subsequent verbatim transcription of data, provides a complete record of the content of the interview. This is a common procedure and most respondents will be agreeable. It enables an analysis of respondents' perspectives based on what they had to say rather than on an interviewer's summaries or paraphrasing. The advantages to respondents can be stressed:

○ It ensures that you will not miss out on any detail that may be important.

○ For busy health professionals, that audio-recording may result in a shorter interview may be a selling point.

○ Audio-recording also allows the researcher to conduct a more effective interview. The interviewer can concentrate on listening to the respondent and ensuring that additional details and clarification are requested for all relevant issues.

○ Assurances of confidentiality must be given. Once data are transcribed the recording should be deleted.

Some notes will be taken in an audio-recorded interview. However, these are minimal and generally act as an aid in the interviewing process, e.g. if a respondent alludes to an event or viewpoint that you believe to be relevant, you may not wish to interrupt at that point, but to make a brief note and continue with the discussion. You can then come back to it and request further detail or explanation.

If a respondent does not wish the interview to be audio-recorded this should not be seen as a problem. Hand notes, as detailed as possible, should be taken instead. The interview may take a bit longer and you can explain that you would like to take careful notes of what he or she says. Immediately after the interview, go through the hand notes and clarify any points where detail is limited or that might later appear unclear. In the analysis these data will be useful, although they cannot be quoted as verbatim responses.

To each interview you should take all the necessary audio-recording equipment with you, including spare batteries, mains adaptor and discs/cassettes. At the start, middle and end of the interview, check that it is being successfully recorded. If, after an interview, you discover that there were problems of which you were unaware, make as detailed hand notes as you can, as soon as possible.

Interviewing is a skilled task. Familiarising yourself with the interview schedule before you attempt any interviews will be invaluable and increase your confidence. If you are new to it you should conduct a small number of pilot interviews just to develop and check your technique. These interviews should also be audio-recorded. You can then play them back and assess your technique for:

○ the use of open questions

○ pacing of the interview and allowing some silence

○ listening skills

○ response to, and follow-up of, issues raised by respondents

○ avoidance of leading questions.

Reliability and validity in interviews

In qualitative research the issues of reliability and validity are addressed in different ways. It is, however, equally important that steps be taken to ensure the quality of the data. Reliability, which refers to the reproducibility of responses, is in some ways not a pertinent issue in qualitative work. The aim is to examine the relevant issues in context. Any inconsistencies in responses should be followed up in the interview and the reasons for these elicited. It should not be assumed that these are 'incorrect'. Explanations should be sought for apparent contradictions so that a detailed understanding of the issues from the perspective of the interviewee is obtained. Thus, it is important that the interviewer pays careful attention to responses, to ensure that all the relevant information is collected during the interview, otherwise difficulties will arise in the data processing and analysis. As the interviewer, the following is the question that you may ask yourself: 'Could I provide a coherent summary of the interviewee's views and reasoning?'

Validity refers to the 'truth' of the data. Some researchers argue that, as long as the interviewer is skilled and attentive in observing the principles of qualitative enquiry (i.e. exercises a sound interviewing technique), the data will have some inherent validity because they should be a true reflection of the respondent's perspectives. Qualitative data are viewed as valuable because they are a product of the views, priorities, experiences, etc. of people on topics of interest to researchers, practitioners and/or policy-makers. However, you must be aware that bias may creep into the data-collection process, e.g. by making assumptions about the respondent, or allowing your own preconceived ideas to colour your questioning and exploration of the issues. Of course it is also important that you are non-leading in the interview and that you can describe the steps you took to avoid influencing the interviewee in his or her responses.

Other factors that can affect the validity of the work and which should be addressed in the planning of the study and information provided are:

○   the location of the interview, e.g. people may feel uncomfortable about raising problems with health services in a pharmacy or other healthcare setting

○   uncertainty about the independence of the researcher, e.g. they may be reluctant to provide detailed accounts of their experiences or concerns if they think that this might get back to their pharmacist, doctor, etc.

○   concerns about confidentiality of data, which may also influence what they are prepared to say.

Further issues about the reliability and validity of qualitative data arise in the data processing and analysis and are discussed in Chapter 5.

Other ways of collecting the data: telephone interviews

One-to-one face-to-face interviews are the most common interview format. However, data may also be gathered by telephone. In general, telephone interviews are more suited to structured questioning than in-depth qualitative work, which requires thoughtful and considered responses. If arranged in advance, at a time convenient for the interviewee, however, they can be successful. These interviews are generally less time-consuming for the researcher, especially if the population is spread over a wide geographical area; they may then enable a larger number of interviews to be conducted within limited time and resources. They present some difficulties too, e.g. the sample members must be individually identifiable and contactable by telephone. In any household, less mobile members may not answer the telephone; in a pharmacy it may be difficult to verify the status of the person to whom you are speaking; a lack of privacy (about which the researcher may be unaware) may affect the frankness of responses.

Interview data may also be collected in group interviews or focus groups.

FOCUS GROUPS/GROUP INTERVIEWS

Focus groups or group interviews are usually considered a qualitative technique. As one-to-one interviews they are conducted by an interviewer, often referred to as the facilitator, with the aid of an interview schedule or guide.

The important difference between one-to-one and group interviews is the interaction between respondents provided by the latter. Thus, commonly, focus groups are employed in exploratory work in which it is believed that the interaction between individuals may stimulate a wide-ranging discussion and generate a comprehensive list of concerns and issues important to respondents. If issues are sensitive, one-to-one interviews may be more effective, if not essential, in providing detailed information. However, if people are prepared to discuss their views and experiences openly, the group setting may provide an opportunity to explore the issues raised by respondents from a range of different perspectives.

Focus groups are generally employed in exploratory work although more structured group techniques (e.g. nominal group technique) have been used in consensus building, often involving groups of 'experts'.

Conducting a focus group

A researcher, or facilitator, is responsible for steering the discussion with the aid of an interview guide. This is usually a semi-structured instrument comprising mainly open questions with a series of prompts or probing questions to extend the discussion. The points raised in response to each open question should be fully explored before moving on to other questions. In response to each point raised, the facilitator should endeavour to elicit contributions from all participants. When promoting discussion of different views and experiences in relation to each issue and in encouraging participation of all members of the group, prompting questions in the interview guide that may be helpful to the facilitator include:

○ Does anyone else share this view?

○ Has anyone had a different experience?

Achieving participation of all group members is a particular challenge of focus group research. Inevitably, in any group there will be more and less vocal members. If the facilitator does not plan and adopt strategies to promote wide participation, the value of group interaction (the reason for choosing this technique in the first place) is lost. As with one-to-one qualitative interviews, and for the same reasons, it is usual, with the permission of all participants, to audio-record the discussion.

A second researcher is also required at the group. Usually this researcher does not take part in the discussion but ensures the effective audio-recording and takes notes about the contributions made by individuals, so that these can be distinguished in the transcripts. Participants could be identified by numbers 1, 2, 3, 4, etc. around the table for this purpose. If contributions cannot be attributed to specific individuals, the extent to which views are shared will be unknown and group interaction, which may be important in interpreting the findings, cannot be taken into account. The second researcher should also take responsibility for administrative tasks, welcoming latecomers, organising refreshments, etc. so that the facilitator can concentrate on ensuring an effective discussion.

In terms of the reliability and validity of the data, many of the principles discussed in relation to one-to-one interviews will apply.

OBSERVATION (PARTICIPANT AND NON-PARTICIPANT)

Participant observation refers to a technique, common in anthropology, in which the researcher lives or participates as a member of the community or group under study. These studies are generally descriptive, confined to single settings and involve the documentation of events or other phenomena in the contexts in which they occur. Participant observation is usually applied as a qualitative technique.

In non-participant observation, the observer is independent of the setting (i.e. an outsider). In pharmacy practice research, non-participant observation is far more common. Non-participant observation has been used in qualitative and quantitative studies, but is more usually employed as a quantitative technique.

Direct observation by a non-participant observer has the benefit that data are 'first hand' rather than relying on individuals' reports of what they do. Sometimes the best way to collect data is to watch what is going on. However, this can present many logistical difficulties and is often not feasible for studies involving large samples.

In quantitative studies, the observer will record details, according to a predetermined schedule, of events or activities as they occur. Often the instrument used will be a structured data-collection form, designed for the study, so that for each event or activity similar details are collected, e.g. details recorded may include the frequency of a particular event or activity, the time, its duration, members of staff involved, other relevant details, etc.

To gather comprehensive data, the researcher must be positioned where they can see and (if necessary) hear what is going on. However, they must also be as unobtrusive as possible and not disruptive to those activities that they are there to document. In many settings this needs careful planning and discussion with staff. If the researcher is not in a position to record all relevant information, this will affect the reliability of the data. If the presence of the researcher affects normal activities or influences the behaviours of those being observed, this undermines the validity of the data. The impact of the presence of the researcher on the activities or people being observed is referred to as the Hawthorne effect. Minimising the Hawthorne effect is a major consideration for these studies. It must be assumed that the researcher will have some impact. The first step to addressing this is to ensure that the researcher is as unobtrusive as possible (while still able to record all relevant information). The second step is to attempt to ascertain in what ways and to what extent the researcher's presence affected the events under study, e.g. some behaviours are more likely to be affected than others; a small amount of undercover observation may be possible for comparative purposes. Alternatively, information may be available from other sources that can be used as an indication of the validity of findings.

Other methods of collecting similar data

Alternative methods include self-reports by individuals of events, e.g. in questionnaires, or by requesting individuals to maintain their own records of events or activities, e.g. by keeping a diary. These methods have the advantage that the researcher does not have to be present for long periods in each setting. Particularly for infrequent events, stationing a researcher on site can be unacceptably time-consuming and expensive, especially if an alternative approach can be found. The disadvantage of depending on others to report the frequency of events or maintain diaries is that reliability cannot be assured (see below). In a questionnaire, people's perceptions or memories of events may not be accurate.

PROSPECTIVE RECORDING OF EVENTS AND DIARIES

Diaries for the reporting of events and activities (referred to above) and time and motion studies are examples of prospective recording of events. For studies involving large samples, or when it is just not feasible for a researcher to be present, participants recruited to the study may be asked to record details of events or their actions. When people are asked to collect data without the researcher being present, steps must be taken to safeguard the quality of the data.

First, the more complicated and labour-intensive the task that participants are asked to undertake, the more likely it is that there will be problems of completeness, reliability and validity. In particular:

○   If events are rare, people can forget that they are supposed to be keeping records.

○   If events are frequent and/or at busy times, maintaining records may be impractical.

○   If data collection extends over a long period, commitment may wane.

In planning the study procedures you should consult with potential participants about the feasibility of the task, the likely problems and how these may be minimised. This may help increase their commitment and observance of the study procedures, and realise their importance. Data-collection forms or diary entries should be quick and easy to complete. Limiting time periods of data collection and the level of detail may help increase reliability. If instructions are clear, it is more likely that they will be closely followed, which will mean that information is more complete. Simple practical steps may make a big difference, such as providing a clipboard for display of the documents, ensuring an appropriate print size, attaching a pen, or in the case of a diary discussing the size of the paper or booklet and its layout.

It is important to check that what you are asking participants to do is acceptable, not too time-consuming or difficult. Study procedures and data quality should be tested in pilot work. During the study it is a good idea to keep in contact with participants to check whether they are experiencing problems in adhering to the study protocol and to address any difficulties as early as possible.

RETROSPECTIVE ANALYSIS OF DATA-SETS MAINTAINED FOR OTHER PURPOSES

Some research objectives can be met by analysis of data already in existence, e.g. databases that are kept for other

purposes (such as routinely maintained prescribing information) or data that have been collected for previous research
(on which you will perform a secondary analysis).

Assuming that either data are in the public domain or
that ethical approval can be obtained, these data-sets can be a
valuable resource. Difficulties can arise for researchers in
retrospectively verifying the completeness of data. Further-
more, although the data-set may be huge, it may not include
all variables pertinent to the objectives of the study, thus
limiting the value of the findings. As the researcher you have
to decide whether these limitations outweigh the benefits of
having a readily accessible data-set.

ANALYSIS OF DOCUMENTS

Analysis of documents should be systematic. This applies to
their identification and selection as well as the analytical
procedures. If the findings are to be generalised, all possible
sources of relevant information should be identified and
material selected that is representative of all of them. Data
processing, coding and analytical procedures should be clear
and consistently applied.

TRIANGULATION AND EVALUATION OF SERVICES

The application of two or more different approaches or
methods within a single study is common in pharmacy practice research. This may be to meet different research objectives or as part of the validation process (see Chapter 2). Some
examples are:

O A series of unstructured or semi-structured interviews sometimes precedes a quantitative study. The two stages may be
independent studies, each scientifically designed with its own
aims and objectives, or the purpose of the first stage may be to
explore the relevant issues to aid the development of a quantitative instrument, such as a questionnaire, for a second
stage.

O Some studies may commence with a quantitative study that is
followed by a more detailed investigation of particular individuals identified in the first stage.

O In terms of validation, observation in a small number of
settings may be used to validate the responses to a questionnaire, or a small number of participants may be inter-
viewed to examine the use of diaries and to speculate on the
probable completeness of data.

O For studies to evaluate services and interventions, see
below.

Evaluating services and interventions

Studies that commonly combine different methods to achieve
a diverse set of research objectives are those that aim to
evaluate a service or intervention. As discussed in Chapter 2,
a new service may be evaluated on a wide range of measures
relating to both processes and outcomes, taking into account
the perspectives of different stakeholders. An evaluation
may:

O include measures of clinical effectiveness, costs, acceptability
to professionals, clients and healthcare organisations, accessibility to clients, and other specific outcomes that the service
was designed to achieve

○   attempt to measure anticipated outcomes against the expectations of the different stakeholders or specific policy objectives

○   as part of the assessment of the feasibility of the service, identify unanticipated problems that arise in its provision.

In addition, the study may include a range of population groups (policy-makers, health professionals, clients), each of which will require a separate sampling strategy, recruitment procedure, data collection method and instrument. Thus, to achieve a comprehensive evaluation, meeting all objectives, a number of different approaches and methods may be required.

CONCLUSION

The range of approaches and methods that may be employed in pharmacy practice and related research to answer important questions is diverse. As all methods have their strengths and weaknesses, for any given study no method may be perfect. The art of choosing the most feasible and effective approach sometimes demands the selection of the best compromise, being aware of its limitations and ensuring that these are addressed as expertly as possible in the study procedures. Potential shortcomings that cannot be resolved must be taken into account when interpreting the study findings.

RS 122.5   B5

RC 46.J6

5

Data processing and analysis

Data collection is followed by data processing and analysis. Data processing comprises those activities required to prepare the data for analysis. Although many tasks will be common to most studies, these activities will depend to some extent on the type of data and the analytical techniques employed; in particular, distinct approaches are associated with quantitative and qualitative research.

QUANTITATIVE RESEARCH

Quantitative studies are those for which the researcher wishes to measure particular phenomena. Examples are establishing the frequency of events, reporting numbers of people involved in certain activities, or ascertaining the proportion of a population who hold a particular view. Researchers may wish to quantify relationships between variables (e.g. examine associations between the characteristics of respondents, the views they may hold and their behaviours). Some studies are designed to test a hypothesis. These will involve the application of probability statistics to measure the differences between groups and the likelihood that the differences represent real differences rather than chance occurrences. Quantitative studies (e.g. survey research) often generate large data-sets, as a result of the number of variables (questions) and/or cases (respondents). In general, questionnaires, structured interviews (i.e. in which a questionnaire is employed in an interview setting), non-participant observation (which involves the gathering of structured data), prospective recording of events and analysis of existing data-sets are methods for which quantitative analytical procedures will be applied.

DATA PROCESSING

Coding frames and coding

The first stage in the processing of quantitative data is the collation of all questionnaires and/or data-collection instruments for coding. Coding of data requires the development of a coding frame. The coding frame consists of specification of codes for all variables (e.g. questions in a questionnaire) and values of (i.e. potential responses to) these variables in the data-set.

As questionnaires generally include a high proportion of closed questions (in which a limited number of response options are provided in the questionnaire), much of the instrument can be pre-coded, i.e. codes can be decided in advance, and the question laid out so that the respondents indicate their response by circling the appropriate code. Open questions require an additional stage in data processing. To these questions the respondents can answer in any way they wish. The coding frame is then usually based on the actual responses made and will often be developed after the data have been collected. From the questionnaires, the researcher will list the different responses that have been given, attempt to group them together and then assign codes. Similar procedures will be followed for other standardised data-collection instruments, e.g. records of observations, diary entries, etc.

Missing data must also be coded. A different code should be allocated to data that are missing because the question was not applicable and for questions not answered for a reason that is unclear (i.e. missing data). In the data analysis it is then possible to include or exclude missing and/or not-applicable cases as appropriate. It is important to be able to state the number of cases for which data are missing.

Codes may also be included for contextual information, situational variables or details of the data collection process, e.g. in interview data, codes may be assigned to enable identification of the interviewer; for data collected in a number of different locations, a code may be used to indicate this. Codes may also be applied to indicate the date of receipt of a returned questionnaire and/or whether it followed the initial or a subsequent mailing. These factors can then be explored in the analysis. A unique code or case number should also be assigned to each respondent (or case) to enable identification.

Coding can be more complicated for questions that allow the respondent to select more than one response (i.e. multiple response items). In the instrument, directions should be clear about how many responses may be selected and whether these should be ranked. For these questions the coding frame must be designed so that the required analyses can be performed. For some analyses, it may be necessary to code each possible response as if it were a separate variable (question).

The coding frame should also include directions for the researchers with regard to the coding procedures, especially how to code ambiguous or unusual responses, e.g. a decision has to be made by the researchers about how a response should be coded if the respondent ticked two boxes. The researchers have to use their judgement in making these decisions. What is important is that these decisions are documented and consistently applied.

The data are coded in accordance with the coding frame, and codes are usually entered directly on to each questionnaire or data collection form.

The reliability of coding should be checked, especially for open questions that can be difficult to interpret and categorise. Detailed instructions in the coding frame are very helpful here. The reliability of the coding procedure can be checked by comparing the codes assigned independently by two researchers to a sample of data. This forms a check of *inter-rater reliability*.

Data entry

Coded data are entered into a database for analysis. A number of statistical packages are available for this. Probably the most commonly used is the Statistical Package for the Social Sciences (SPSS). This program allows a wide range of simple and complex statistical procedures which are appropriate for pharmacy practice and related research. Some databases are limited in the analytical procedures that are possible. It is important to know what procedures will be needed and to check that the software has the capacity to meet them.

Data entry is a mechanical task, but it is important. The validity of the analysis depends on its accuracy. Care with data entry and systematic checking is fundamental. A single incorrect entry can result in having to repeat whole sets of analyses. Conversely, if the coding and data entry procedures are carried out with care and appropriate checking, the analysis should be smooth. The process of checking for, identifying and rectifying inaccuracies is referred to as 'cleaning' the data.

Approaching the analysis

Software packages for statistical analysis of quantitative (e.g. survey) data are very powerful. They offer the possibility of a great variety of procedures and manipulations of data. A danger arises, therefore, that if you perform a large number of tests of relationships between variables you will inevitably chance upon some statistically significant associations, e.g. if a 0.05 level of statistical significance is selected, as is conventional, this means that a relationship between variables is assumed to be real if there is a 95% probability that it would not have occurred by chance, i.e. there is a 1 in 20 chance that the association is spurious. In other words, for every 20 tests performed, one statistically significant result would be expected even if there were no systematic relationships between variables in the data-set.

Data analysis in which researchers test for associations between variables in the data-set until they find them are sometimes referred to as 'fishing expeditions'. To avoid the possibility of misleading findings, statisticians advise that the analysis should be planned in advance according to the specific study objectives.

A second consideration when approaching the data analysis is to be aware of the limitations of the data. Non-random sampling procedures, small data-sets, poorly constructed questions, unreliable responses, missing values, etc. all limit the validity of the data. It is important to be realistic about the quality of the data. In survey research it is well recognised that some questions may be problematic, affecting the validity of the responses. If, during the data collection or data processing, it becomes apparent that some questions presented difficulties, consideration should be given to the exclusion of these from the analysis.

Software packages for statistical analysis place a huge range of complex and powerful procedures at the disposal of the researcher. Many are simple to perform in that programs are often menu driven. However, this simplicity can mask the complexity of the procedures, most of which rest on complicated assumptions about the structure of the data-set. If these assumptions do not apply, the procedures may be invalid and meaningless. Ensuring that the data conform to the necessary assumptions requires considerable understanding and expertise. Failure to check that these assumptions are not violated can result in a real danger of performing inappropriate analyses, leading to incorrect conclusions.

Selection of statistical procedures for descriptive studies

Data analysis will be governed by the study objectives. For descriptive studies, analyses commonly include the following:

O   Procedures to summarise the characteristics of large data-sets, e.g. analysis of frequencies, calculations of means, medians, standard deviations, etc. These are sometimes referred to as descriptive statistics.

O   Investigations of associations between the variables in the data set, e.g. cross- tabulations, chi-squared (χ^2) tests, t-tests, Mann–Whitney U tests, correlation.

○   More complex investigations of association between variables can be performed using multivariate methods (procedures that are performed on data relating to three or more variables simultaneously). These procedures include regression, analysis of variance, factor analysis, some modelling procedures, etc.

In the selection of the appropriate analytical procedures, the characteristics of the data in terms of, first, the type of variable and, second, the distribution of the values as parametric (usually normally distributed) or non-parametric (distribution-free) must be determined.

Types of variable

In quantitative research, data relating to each variable may be nominal (in which a value or code is assigned to each of the possible responses which have no inherent order or ranking, e.g. male = 1, female = 2; or yes = 1, no = 2), ordinal (where codes are applied, and the value of the code represents increasing value of the variable, e.g. occasionally = 1, sometimes = 2, often = 3) or interval/ratio (where the value or code represents a true value, e.g. total serum cholesterol or the number of prescription medicines currently prescribed for an individual).

Parametric and non-parametric data

This refers to the distribution of values for any variable. Probability statistics used in health services research are commonly based on the normal distribution. For the application of these techniques to be valid there is an underlying assumption that the data are normally distributed. For many variables, especially various biochemical and physiological measures (e.g. height, weight, blood pressure in a population), this is generally the case. However, for other variables this may not be so. Commonly, in health services and pharmacy practice research data will be non-parametric, e.g. the number of prescription drugs regularly taken by a population would not be expected to be normally distributed (a high proportion of the population may take none or one, and progressively fewer take larger numbers). Journey times to a pharmacy may also be skewed, with the majority of the population living within a very short distance whereas small numbers have very extended journey times. If data are not normally distributed, non-parametric procedures should be employed.

Descriptive procedures and summary statistics

Often the first stage of analysis in a descriptive study is to obtain frequency data on most or all of the variables in the data-set. This will provide descriptive information on all respondents according to their responses to the questions, e.g. the number of male and female respondents, their age group, work location, views on particular issues, number of prescription-related problems recorded, etc. according to the questionnaire. This information can be supplemented by summary statistics. Rather than list all the values, reporting the mean or median values or a measure of the spread of the values may be helpful.

If data are normally distributed, the mean value (arithmetic average = sum of all values/number of cases) can be reported. In normally distributed data the mean and the median will be similar. The median (middle value) is used in non-parametric data. This provides an indication of the value that is characteristic of an 'average' member of the population. In data-sets in which a small proportion of the population report unusually high values, this will be reflected in a higher population mean. The median value may then be a more useful reflection of a typical population value for a variable that is skewed by the presence of a small number of unusually low or high values.

Measures of spread of data include standard deviation (for normally distributed data), maximum and minimum values, and interquartile ranges. If the data are normally distributed, the standard deviation is very informative because two-thirds of cases will lie within one standard deviation of the mean and 95% will lie within two standard deviations.

Investigating associations between categorical variables

If the data-set is sufficiently large, associations between different variables in a data-set can be investigated, e.g. age of respondent and number of prescribed medicines, or location of pharmacy and workload. Selection of the best procedure is governed by the type of data (as nominal, ordinal or interval/ratio) and the distribution of the values (as normal or non-normal).

Nominal data (categorical data)

Cross-tabulation of data enables documentation of the number of cases according to pre-determined categories. A table is constructed that categorises each case according to the response to each of two variables, thus forming a cell structure. A χ^2 test may then be performed to indicate whether the number of cases in each cell departs from that which would be expected if there were no association between the variables, e.g. to investigate whether male or female pharmacists were more or less likely to respond to a questionnaire, a χ^2 test would compare the actual number of male and female respondents and non-respondents with the numbers that would be expected if there were no systematic differences between them. From the χ^2 statistic, the probability that the responses represent a systematic difference between the groups can be ascertained.

For the χ^2 test to be valid there should be an expected frequency of at least five cases in each cell. Also a correction factor is required for small (2×2, i.e. one degree of freedom) tables. Care is required with large tables (i.e. variables for which there are a large number of categories/values) because the test does not specify where any differences lie.

Ordinal data and non-normally distributed interval data

Non-parametric procedures are used to investigate the possible statistical significance of differences between groups when data are either ordinal or do not form a normal distribution. To compare data from two groups (e.g. male and female respondents) a Mann–Whitney U test is commonly performed. This is based on rankings of all cases according to the variable of interest. The ranks for the two groups are then compared and assessed to establish the likelihood that the differences in the ranks could have occurred by chance. The Kruskal–Wallis test is a similar procedure employed when more than two groups are being compared.

Interval/ratio data that are normally distributed

To compare two groups of respondents on a normally distributed variable, a t-test can be performed. This compares the mean values for each group and, based on normal distribution theory, assesses whether the difference is likely to have occurred by chance or to represent a real difference between the two groups. Analysis of variance (ANOVA) can be used to assess differences between more than two groups.

Associations between two ordered or continuous variables

Correlation is used to assess the relationship between two ordered or continuous variables, i.e. the extent to which an increase in one variable is associated with an increase in the other (e.g. the extent to which blood pressure rises with age). Non-parametric procedures (e.g. Spearman's correlation) are used for ordinal or non-normally distributed data. Simple linear correlation, e.g. based on the theory of least squares, can be used for normally distributed data. Before the calculation of a correlation coefficient, a scatter plot should be drawn to assess the appropriateness of the procedure, e.g. there may be a relationship between the values of the variables that is not linear and therefore would not be identified by this procedure.

Multivariate procedures

The procedures outlined above involve the analysis of data relating to two variables at a time. These bivariate procedures are commonly employed in the initial investigations of relationships between variables. Procedures that analyse data relating to three or more variables simultaneously are referred to as multivariate. Multivariate procedures assume that the variables will be interrelated, i.e. that a change in the value of one variable will be accompanied by a change in the value of others. In these circumstances it is seen as appropriate to adopt a multivariate approach to the analysis. Computer software provides opportunities for researchers to undertake complex and exciting procedures in the analysis of their data. The common packages designed for the analysis of quantitative (especially survey) data offer a wide range of multivariate procedures.

It is beyond the scope of this text to detail the wide range of multivariate procedures that may be performed. However, by way of an overview, multivariate procedures are sometimes classified as dependence methods, in which one or more variables are identified as the variables of interest (dependent variable(s)). Analytical procedures then focus on explaining changes in the values of the dependent variables in terms of others, i.e. independent variables. Examples of these procedures are multiple regression, discriminant analysis and multivariate analysis of variance (MANOVA).

Regression is one of the most common, more complex procedures used in the analysis of quantitative data. This is a technique to identify variables (independent variables) that are predictive of a variable of interest (dependent variable), e.g. to identify factors that are predictive of the level of consumption of non-prescription medicines. Logistic regression is employed when the dependent variable takes on two nominal values. Discriminant analysis may provide an alternative to logistic regression. In this procedure, independent variables are combined into a new variable that distinguishes between individuals in terms of the dependent variable. MANOVA is similar to ANOVA in that it assesses differences between groups, but on the basis of more than one dependent variable.

Other procedures are classified as interdependence methods. These are where the variables are analysed as a single interrelated set, none of which is designated as dependent or otherwise of particular importance for the purposes of the analysis. Factor and cluster analyses are examples of these procedures.

Factor analysis has been widely used in survey work in pharmacy practice, especially in studies of people's beliefs and attitudes. It is a data-reduction technique that is used to reduce a larger number of variables to a smaller number of underlying dimensions or factors. Cluster analysis enables individuals or cases to be distinguished or grouped (into clusters) in terms of other variables in the data-set.

Multivariate analyses are complicated. A limited understanding of the underlying mathematics and assumptions of these procedures risks their inappropriate use. Their availability in common software packages for the analysis of survey data can lead to their application to data-sets that were not designed with these procedures in mind. Great care must be taken to ensure the validity of their application.

Inferential statistics

Much research is based on data derived from a sample rather than the whole population. Confidence intervals enable the extrapolation of findings, based on the sample estimates, to the population from which the sample was drawn (assuming that a probability sampling procedure was followed). The calculation of confidence intervals is based on normal distribution theory. Thus, for normally distributed data, the width of the confidence intervals provides an indication of how accurate the estimate (derived from the sample) is likely to be when applied to the study population. A confidence interval (conventionally 95%) consists of two values, one of which will be below and the other above the sample mean. Thus, although not able to state the precise population mean value, the researcher can be 95% sure that it is between these two values.

Scales and reliability

Instruments to investigate people's views and beliefs commonly comprise a series of questions or items to which participants respond on a Likert scale (strongly agree, agree, neither agree nor disagree, disagree, strongly disagree). Frequency analysis will usually be the first stage of the analysis of the data. As a result of the non-linearity of the Likert scale, the validity of any scaling procedure (e.g. summing scores on different items) must be assured before it is used. Factor analysis is sometimes used to identify components of these beliefs or views. By contrast, assumptions of linearity are made in respect of visual analogue scales. Cronbach's α is a measure of reliability which is commonly applied to assess the internal consistency of the items of a scale.

Statistical analysis in intervention studies

As with descriptive studies, the first step in the analysis may be to present frequency data to enable examination of the important characteristics of, and differences between, the data-sets. However, in analysing the data from intervention or experimental studies, additional procedures are employed which focus on testing for statistically significant differences between the groups (intervention and control).

It would be unlikely in any study for the results from two groups to be identical. Statistical procedures are used to assess whether the differences between the intervention and control groups represent real differences between the two data-sets or whether they probably just occurred by chance statistical significance are conducted.

A statistical significance test is based on the assumption that the two data-sets (intervention and control) could have come from the 'same population'. Two samples from a population may not be identical, but they should be similar. Given the similarities (or differences) between the two sets of data (intervention and control group), what is the chance that both come from the same population? If, based on statistical theory, the differences between the two samples are such that the likelihood that they are from the same population is very small, we may decide to accept that there is a real difference between the two groups. By convention, in much research P values of less than 0.05 (or 5%) are often taken as conferring statistical significance, i.e. there is a less than 5% probability that the differences between the two groups would have occurred by chance.

When reporting the results, it is usual to report summary statistics for each of the groups on all the comparator variables. This will indicate the size of differences between the intervention and control groups, as well as establishing whether or not the difference is statistically significant.

QUALITATIVE RESEARCH

Data processing and analysis in qualitative research employ a very different range of techniques from quantitative research. Small numbers of respondents and detailed contextual information are a feature of the data-sets of these studies. Data are commonly verbatim transcripts of semi-structured or in-depth interviews, transcripts of discussions of focus groups or (less commonly in pharmacy practice research) detailed field notes of observations by researchers. Analysis of qualitative data is a highly skilled task. There are numerous texts dedicated to the description and rationale of possible approaches and procedures.

Approaches to data processing and analysis

The approach to data processing and analysis will depend on the study objectives, in particular the extent to which the research follows purist principles of qualitative enquiry (e.g. unstructured interviews), as opposed to a more structured framework determined by the researcher's pre-set agenda. Thus, the goals of the research may range from the development of theories or hypotheses to explain phenomena of interest, to the provision of detailed descriptions of respondents' views or experiences with regard to specific situations or events. These goals will influence the approach to data collection, processing and analysis.

All qualitative studies require observance of principles of qualitative enquiry such that the data are an objective and comprehensive reflection of the issues of relevance to the respondents. All require data processing and analytical techniques that result in a full and accurate representation of the perspectives of respondents.

Grounded theory methodology is an example of a more purist approach of qualitative enquiry. This is an inductive theory-building process that allows ideas and explanations of phenomena to emerge from the data in the context of natural settings. Through repeated data collection, processing and analysis, theory is developed, refined and verified.

Procedures of data processing and analysis

The first stage in the data processing of qualitative material is generally verbatim transcription of interviews. This can be a very time-consuming task. One 20-minute interview will usually take several hours to transcribe. A lengthy focus group discussion may take several days. Contextual data from field notes may also be included.

The development of coding frames and the coding of data are employed in most qualitative studies. Thus, devising a coding frame is commonly the next step of data processing after transcription of data.

In qualitative research the structure and content of the coding frame will be derived from the data, i.e. it is based on the issues, descriptions, explanations, etc. provided by respondents. Thus, unlike some quantitative studies, in which coding frames can be developed at the same time as the instrument, in qualitative work development of the coding frame has to follow data collection. The first step is for the researchers to familiarise themselves with the data (often achieved during transcription) and to identify a thematic framework that covers all the issues raised by respondents. Identification of principal themes from within the data-set and their organisation into a framework (which may just be a list of distinct topic areas) may form the primary coding structure.

The primary coding framework for semi-structured interviews may be derived from an interview schedule that will have been devised to influence the direction of the discussion. In other cases, the objectives of the study may provide a framework for the primary coding procedure.

These primary codes can then be applied to the data-set to enable identification of all data relevant to each of these themes or topic areas within the data-set. During the application of these primary codes to the data, some additional themes or topics may emerge, necessitating some revision of the primary coding frame. These may be the identification of new issues (that do not fit existing codes) which therefore require new codes, or the division of some themes into distinct topic areas requiring additional codes.

After identification of the principal themes, the researcher embarks on a more detailed examination of data within each of these areas. This may involve the development of a separate coding structure for data relating to each of the principal themes. These themes may be subdivided, with different codes used to distinguish specific situational factors or types of explanation provided by the respondents. The researcher may also wish to build into the coding structure the capacity to cross-link issues, situational factors, explanations, etc. relevant to more than one principal theme.

The coding structure, to some extent, will evolve as the analysis proceeds. It must enable the organisation of the data so as to facilitate its examination and interpretation. As the analysis proceeds, new questions or hypotheses may arise which the researcher will want to investigate. This may lead to the development of a further level of coding to enable identification of all material that may be relevant. Thus, in qualitative work, data processing and analysis are likely to be integrated. Development of coding frames and coding of transcripts form part of the analytical process. As the analysis proceeds, the coding frame may be developed further, i.e. coding and analysis are sometimes interactive. After modifications and refinements to the coding frame or the development of a new code, this revised coding frame must then be applied systematically to all cases. This can mean recoding all data.

Coding and analysis of qualitative data are often an involved and complicated procedure, sometimes with continual reassessment. Management of the data requires good organisation on the part of the researcher. To assist in this a number of computer packages are available. These may be a useful aid in the management of large data-sets, to facilitate the retrieval of data once coded; sifting through data by hand to extract the relevant sections can be time-consuming. They may also be helpful in validation processes, e.g. by efficient identification of all instances in which a topic was raised.

Reliability and validity in qualitative work

Analysis of qualitative data (as interviewing) is a skilled task. Interpretation by the researcher is an important part of the analytical process. Thus, steps must be taken to ensure the reliability of procedures and the validity of findings. Two or more researchers may be involved in the development of the coding frame, possibly independently devising their own structures, which are then compared.

As with quantitative work, codes must be consistently applied to the data. As a check on the reliability of the coding process, it is common for this to be undertaken by two researchers independently for a sample of the transcripts. Any discrepancies in the coding must be examined and the coding frame or guidelines for its use revised to ensure its consistent application.

In qualitative work it is important that *all* issues and perspectives raised by respondents are included in the analysis. A topic may be raised only once and it could be that it is of minor importance. On the other hand, it may be that it is a result of particular situational or circumstantial factors, and as such becomes an important issue in the context of the data-set.

The validity of the results (i.e. the extent to which they are a true representation of phenomena under study) must also be assured. There are many opportunities for bias to colour the analytical process. A number of approaches can be employed to validate research findings:

○   In the course of the analysis, the researcher may attempt to use the data to argue a viewpoint contradictory to the tentative conclusions or theories, i.e. the researcher will (as the devil's advocate) look for specific examples in the data that do not fit with his or her hypothesis or conclusions.

○   After data analysis, the researcher may collect additional data to verify a hypothesis or ask the original participants to comment on the extent to which they believe the findings accurately represent their perspectives.

○   Researchers may compare their findings with those of other studies (in the literature) or relevant theory to assess the extent to which they are consistent.

A systematic and scientific approach to the analysis of qualitative data is of paramount importance to the research. Sound methodological principles and strategies must be rigorously observed if the findings are to be dependable.

Focus groups

In general the principles of qualitative analysis discussed above will apply to focus group data. It is the group interaction that provides an added dimension and distinguishes the analytical process. As for one-to-one interviews, the first stage in the processing of data will be verbatim transcriptions of the group discussions. It is important that in these transcriptions all contributions are attributed to the correct participant. In the analysis, this will enable the researcher to trace and compare the views, perspectives and experiences of individual participants, and also investigate whether and how the views of individuals changed during the course of the discussion.

CONCLUSION

The approaches to, and procedures of, data processing and analysis in quantitative and qualitative research differ greatly. However, observance of sound methodological principles and care in maintaining a rigorous approach are essential. Without this, all stages of data processing and analysis are open to practices that may undermine the reliability and validity of the work. A careful and thorough approach (especially in qualitative studies) can be time-consuming; however, it also facilitates a smooth-running analysis, a rewarding path of discovery, and findings in which you have confidence.

6

Writing up and disseminating the findings

After undertaking an original research project, writing it up and disseminating the findings are an important part of the research process. If you have some interesting results that you believe to be valuable, you will want to ensure that these reach a wider audience. For yourself it is also a recognition of your efforts. Funding bodies will be reluctant to provide resources for research unless they are convinced that the findings will have an application and value. Apart from writing up the project in part fulfilment of a degree, opportunities for wider dissemination could be sought.

WRITING THE PROJECT REPORT

Writing up the report is generally seen as a final stage of any research project. However, it is a good plan not to leave this entirely until the end. Of course, it is not possible to write up the results or discussion until the work is just about complete, but the introduction and methods can be commenced at an earlier stage. For most projects the final weeks can be quite pressurised. Inevitably, throughout the study you will have more and less busy times. Typically, at the start of the project you may have to wait for ethical approval or permission from other bodies. During data collection you may be dependent on the availability of others before you can proceed. You should consider this waiting time as valuable, enabling you to undertake the literature survey and prepare the introduction to your project.

During those times when the study is under way, but you have to wait for the decisions and cooperation of others, you can commence the writing of your methodology and method. It is a good time to do it, when the details about decisions on all aspects of study procedures, preparation of documentation, development of instruments, dealings with ethics committees, liaison with others, etc. are still fresh in your mind. Also, it is an opportunity to take before you become busy completing other aspects of the work.

The project report will usually be very detailed. If the project was undertaken in part fulfilment of the requirements of a degree, there may be guidelines about the content, presentation, length, style of referencing, etc. of the report. However, it will usually comprise the following sections:

- Title page
- Acknowledgements
- Summary or abstract
- Contents, including lists of tables and figures
- Introduction with a statement of the aims and objectives
- Methods
- Results
- Discussion
- Conclusion (and recommendations)
- References
- Appendices

Title page

The title page includes the title of the project, the name of the author and their affiliation/position, the institution from which the research was carried out and the date of completion. If the research was conducted as part of the requirement for a degree programme, this is usually also stated.

The acknowledgements

The acknowledgements are an opportunity for the researcher to thank anyone who helped in the research. This may include people who provided guidance or advice on any part of the study, people who helped in identifying and contacting respondents, anyone who assisted in the data collection and, last but not least, the participants themselves. This last group cannot be mentioned by name, because anonymity must be preserved, but they are usually the most important people in any study. At this point any funding body should also be acknowledged.

The summary or abstract

This is generally one or two pages in length. Even though it appears at the beginning of the report it is often one of the last sections to be written. It provides a brief overview of the background to the study, the objectives, the main methods used, and important findings and conclusions. This abstract is important. It should provoke the reader into reading the rest of the report. It may also be the section from which any reviewers obtain their first impressions.

The contents page

This is often drafted soon after beginning the report. It provides the researcher with a framework for writing. However, because it requires pagination, completing the contents page will be one of the final tasks. The contents page may be followed by lists of tables and figures.

The four sections

The introduction (with a statement of aims and objectives), methods, results and discussion form the main body of the report. The structure and content of each of these sections invariably require careful thought. The information should be presented in a very straightforward and logical way so that it is easy for the reader to follow. However, all the relevant information must be included. Some general guidance for each of these sections is provided below.

Introduction

The introduction should explain to the reader why the study has been undertaken. It will usually include a review of the literature identifying other studies relevant to the research area. It should include some critical evaluation of these works, in terms of their strengths and weaknesses (e.g. comments on how a study was done, whether the topic was comprehensively addressed, what questions it left unanswered or what new issues were raised). Reference should also be made to relevant policy documents or directions in health service provision, professional agendas or practice developments that will demonstrate why the research is important and topical.

After reading the introduction the reader should understand the background to the study and be able to see how the work will add to existing research literature and/or provide important information for specific policy objectives.

The introduction often ends with a statement of the aims and objectives of the project.

Methods

In writing this section attention should be paid to both the methodology and the methods. The section provides an explanation and justification for the methods chosen (i.e. the *methodology*) and a detailed description of the actual *methods* used.

The methods selected depend on the objectives of the study. There may be a number of possible ways of obtaining the data required for each objective. Each will have its advantages and disadvantages in terms of feasibility, efficiency, costs, reliability, ethical problems, etc. The reasons for choosing particular approaches and methods should be discussed, recognising the pros and cons of each and justifying your decisions. This should be done for all stages of the method (e.g. sampling strategy, methods of data collection, development of instruments, procedures for validation, etc.).

Separate sections of the methods may describe each of the following:

○ Preliminary fieldwork and pilot studies

○ Ethical approval, obtaining permission from other bodies

○ Sampling strategy and procedures

○   Recruitment of participants

○   Development of the instruments and data-collection methods

○   Data processing and analysis.

It is important to demonstrate to the reader that the methods were robust, acceptable to participants and well tested. Preliminary fieldwork that informed decisions about the methodology should be reported. Any revisions to the procedures or instruments as a result of the pilot work should be detailed. Thus, it is important to describe how you selected and recruited your sample, the follow-up of non-responders, the steps taken to ensure the reliability of validity of procedures and results, etc.

Copies of any questionnaires, data-collection forms, letters of recruitment, information to participants, consent forms, etc. can be included in the appendices.

Results

The content and structure of this section will be governed by the study objectives. For some studies, sections corresponding to results relating to each of the objectives may provide a suitable framework. If a questionnaire or semi-structured interview schedule were used you could feel that presentation of the results could sensibly follow the question order. In a qualitative study, broad themes identified during the analysis of data may provide a logical way of organising the results section. The length of the results section will vary markedly between studies. For some quantitative studies, the findings can be effectively reported in a few tables with minimal supporting text. Conversely, qualitative work may require detailed discussion of respondents' perspectives on a wide range of issues, possibly supported by verbatim quotations.

The results section will often commence with a report of the number of participants, and the response rates. A description of participants should be provided, e.g. age, sex, location of work, socioeconomic background, aspects of drug use, etc. and any other characteristics relevant to the study. Any available information on non-responders should be reported together, if possible, with a comparison of responders and non-responders. This will enable the reader to assess the probable representativeness of the sample. If relevant information is available, it may be possible to compare some of the characteristics of the sample with those of the wider population.

Quantitative studies

In reporting the findings in quantitative studies, especially frequency data, tables, bar charts, histograms or pie charts can improve the presentation and aid the interpretation of the results. When these are used the accompanying text need not repeat the information in these tables and figures, but can be used to draw attention to important features, comment on and explain any apparent inconsistencies, etc. The text can also be used to report and describe any associations between variables, and to summarise the findings in relation to each study objective.

Qualitative studies

In qualitative work the results and discussion sections are sometimes combined. This can be helpful to the researcher because data analysis is to some extent an interpretative process in which later stages of the analysis build on earlier ones. Points raised in discussion (theoretical perspectives or findings from the literature) may have informed and directed the analysis. In these cases, by combining the two sections it makes it easier to explain the rationale for the analysis and enables you to describe the results in the context of your theoretical framework, e.g. if you wished to examine ways in which your findings support existing theories or hypotheses in the literature, you may have constructed your analysis to enable this investigation. It may be easier to incorporate a discussion of ways in which your data do or do not support this earlier work when presenting your results rather than having separate results and discussion sections, which can result in a lot of repetition.

When combining the results and discussion sections, it can be difficult to ensure that it is always clear to the reader which is which. The combined results/discussion section will comprise the results of your study, discussion points identified in the literature (including results of other studies and/or theoretical perspectives), and your own thoughts on your findings (including bringing the results and discussion together).

In qualitative work verbatim quotations taken directly from the transcripts are sometimes used in the results section. This is only possible for data that are audio-recorded and transcribed verbatim. As the aim of qualitative work is usually to present issues from the perspective of respondents, use of their words to illustrate the findings is seen as logical. However, the rationale for the selection of quotes must be clear. A quotation may be selected to represent, in context, a typical viewpoint or to demonstrate a common problem experienced by respondents. A series of quotes may be used to illustrate a range of viewpoints or experiences, or perhaps to portray extreme cases. Quotations must not be a substitute for analysis and critical thought on the part of the researcher. It is easy to find many interesting quotes, but it can be very challenging to embark on an in-depth analysis and interpretation of the data. Quotes should be selected to illustrate your findings and enhance the reader's insights into the issues. However, in terms of presentation of the results, their use should be seen as secondary and kept to a minimum. It is also conventional to attribute each quote to a respondent. It should be possible for the reader to see which quotations were attributable to the same respondent. Sometimes further information may be provided on relevant characteristics of the respondent; of course anonymity must be preserved.

Qualitative studies generally involve small numbers of respondents, who are purposively selected. Thus, reporting of numbers or proportions of respondents who hold particular views is usually not the intention. However, in some studies, it may be appropriate to inform the reader when a view was universally held or whether an issue was raised by only one individual. This information may provide insights into situational factors or contexts that might give rise to particular phenomena. Qualitative studies may aim to provide possible explanations for phenomena, e.g. a legitimate question may be: 'Could a particular experience or problem result from certain identifiable factors?' Thus, in qualitative studies the reporting of numbers of respondents holding particular views is sometimes helpful and justified.

As a general rule, in the results section of a qualitative study, all issues raised by respondents should be included. Points raised by only one respondent are not necessarily less important. These issues may be pertinent to situational factors that were unique to that particular respondent. If a purposive sampling procedure was employed, there may be

only one such individual in the sample, but similar situations
may be replicated in the wider population.

Discussion

The content of the discussion will be determined by the study
objectives and results. However, a few general thoughts will
be relevant to most studies.

The discussion can be a reiteration of the results, but it
must not be. Avoiding repetition of the results (to facilitate
their discussion) can be difficult. Perhaps the best way to
avoid this is to have a clear alternative agenda for the discussion. The results should be taken as read, the discussion
focusing on their implications, e.g. depending on the objectives and topic area of the study, the following thoughts may
assist you in developing a framework for the discussion:

○   The specific objectives of the study: comment on the extent to
which these were met and the implications of specific findings
for each objective.

○   The literature, including previous studies and/or theoretical
perspectives: relate your findings to those of other researchers. Relevant work will have been identified during the
literature review at the start of the study. Depending on the
duration of your project, it may be necessary to update your
review, to check for more recent work. Consider how your
work builds upon, extends or contradicts existing literature
on the subject. When comparing your findings with those of
others, you should not just report any similarities and differences, but also comment on how any inconsistencies might be
explained.

○   The policy context: if the objective or topic of study has direct
(or indirect) relevance for some aspect of health/pharmacy/

drug use policy. The findings of the study may enable recommendations to be made.

○ The methodological limitations of the study: these should be acknowledged. Suggestions as to how they might be overcome and what implications they may have for the results should be discussed. You should ask the question: 'Given the limitations of the study, are the conclusions really justified?'

You should make it clear to the reader what your work adds to the literature in the field and why it is important or valuable. You should not leave it to readers to work out these things for themselves. The discussion may end with a conclusion and possibly recommendations for pharmacy, healthcare and/or future research.

References

In listing the references, consistency and completeness are of great importance. It is best to use a standard procedure right from the start, such as the Harvard or Vancouver systems. Most journals use one or other of these:

○ The Harvard system includes the names of the author(s) and date of publication in the text. The full citations are then listed alphabetically in the reference section. If there are more than two authors, generally only the first will appear in the text followed by *et al*. The names of all authors will be cited in the reference section. Where there is reference to more than one publication in any year by an author (or the same authors), the suffix a, b, c, etc. follows the date in the text and also in the reference section.

○ The Vancouver system is a numbering system. In the text numbers are used sequentially at each point to be referenced. The reference section then lists in numerical order the full references in order of appearance in the text.

From the early stages of the project, when undertaking the literature review or preliminary fieldwork, you should keep full notes of all your references and other sources (including personal communications). If at a later date you discover that a reference is inaccurate or incomplete it can be very time-consuming and sometimes difficult to trace the original article or source, and this is often at a time when you are very busy completing your project.

You should keep the following records of all references and other sources as you go:

○ Journal articles: names with initials of all authors, year of publication, title of article, full title of journal, volume number, first and last page numbers.

○ Books: names with initials of all authors, year of publication, title of book, place of publication, publisher.

○ Book chapters in an edited (as opposed to authored) book: the author(s) of the chapter with their initials, the chapter number, title of the chapter and first and last page numbers; the names with initials of the editor(s), year of publication, the title of the book, place of publication, publisher.

○ Policy document or document from other public or private body: names with initials of all authors (which may be an organisation or individuals on behalf of an organisation), year of publication, title of document, place of publication, publisher.

○ Website: name of organisation, date of publication or date information accessed, title of article (if applicable), web address.

○ Personal communications: names/affiliations of individuals, names of organisations as appropriate and dates.

Appendices

The appendices should be numbered according to the order in which they are referred to in the project report. They may include copies of letters sent to potential participants, information leaflets/consent forms, questionnaires, interview schedules, data-collection forms and any other study instruments or documentation that may be of interest to the reader. Complete transcripts of interviews (anonymised, of course) can also be included. In some cases, additional, usually more detailed, analyses appear in the appendices, especially when these may be of interest only to specialist readers, be supportive of the procedures reported in the main text or peripheral to the main objectives of the study.

When a maximum word count is prescribed for a project write-up or paper, this often excludes the title page, contents pages, abstract, references and appendices.

PRESENTING THE PROJECT TO A LOCAL AUDIENCE

It is common for research to be presented in the first instance to a local audience. This may be to fellow students who have also been conducting their own projects, members of the department or institution in which the work was conducted, and/or to any individuals who assisted with the work or with a particular interest in the field.

Oral presentations

The level of detail to be included will depend on the length of time available. As a general rule you should aim to leave time for questions and discussion at the end, e.g. in a 15-minute slot, prepare a 10-minute presentation, allowing 5 minutes for discussion. In a 30-minute slot, a 20-minute presentation with 10 minutes for discussion would be appropriate. If you have 45–60 minutes in total you could leave 15–20 minutes for discussion. You should rehearse your talk to familiarise yourself with the points that you wish to make (especially if these include explanations of relatively complex phenomena or procedures) and check that it falls within the time limits.

Oral presentations of research (whether to a local audience or at an international conference) are usually short. If you have spent several weeks, months or even years working on a research project, it will be a challenge to convey your important messages successfully in a limited time. You should also remember that in many cases your audience will be listening to a series of presentations, possibly on varying topics, in a relatively short period. The talk must be well organised, easy to follow, kept as simple as possible while still maintaining the detail and depth required to describe the work accurately and assure the audience of its scientific validity.

Thus, the material to be included must be carefully selected. In a large project you may opt to focus on a single objective rather than attempt to cover all aspects of the work. If you decide to do this, your intention must be made clear to the audience and sufficient background and description of methods must be included. It may be at the results stage that you home in on specific aspects.

The presentation will usually be structured as: introduction, methods, results and discussion/conclusions, all of which will necessarily be brief.

The purpose of the introduction is to inform the reader of the reasons for undertaking the work. A few minutes at the start of the talk may be devoted to describing the problems to be addressed, highlighting any relevant policy issues and/or existing literature on the subject. The introduction often ends with a statement of the aims and objectives of the project. It should be clear how these will contribute to the subject area under study.

A description of the methods will then follow. This should include some justification of why particular procedures were selected and the acknowledgement of any important shortcomings (as well as the strengths). The results of any study must be interpreted in the context of the methods used. Although you do have to be relatively brief, the audience must have some understanding of the methodological approach so that they can come to some independent assessment and interpretation of the results.

The results are usually the most important part of the presentation. These must be well organised and clearly presented. You may commence the results section with an overview of what you are going to present, e.g. you may present the findings relating to each objective in turn. Or you may start with an overview of the main findings and then focus in more detail on selected issues.

It is important to be realistic about the range, detail and depth of information that can be included in the time available. You may have to be selective about what you can include. If graphs or figures are to be used, you must leave sufficient time for explanation of what they show and for the audience to make sense of the material for themselves.

The talk will usually finish with a discussion of points that you feel are important, conclusions relating to the study objectives and/or policy implications of the findings. You may have particular issues that you wish to highlight for discussion. Depending on your audience (e.g. if it includes people with particular expertise or experience) you may request their thoughts on specific aspects of the study procedures or findings. Thus, to some extent you can control the direction of the discussion if you wish.

Attention should also be paid to the presentation of material. Slides should be well laid out, and not congested with too much material. The size of print should be such that text, graphs and figures can easily be read from the back of the room. When presenting you should stand so that you do not obstruct the audience's view of the screen. The number of slides should be appropriate to the length of the talk and the complexity of the material, e.g. you could aim for an average of one slide for every 1–2 minutes of your talk.

Poster presentations

These are a common alternative to oral presentations. At a poster session, the authors stay next to their poster and are ready to discuss their work or answer any questions. Many of the principles discussed above in relation to oral presentations will apply when preparing a poster. Posters, also, are often structured into introduction, methods, results and discussion sections. Material under each of these headings must similarly be carefully selected. In terms of the level of detail, range of issues, etc. you should bear in mind that people may be viewing many posters in a single session, and therefore will spend no more that a few minutes at each. Poster sessions are often quite relaxed and informal. You should aim to convey only a few simple messages in the body of the poster. Including too much complex detail may be offputting. You will be on hand to provide more information should this be requested. You could also prepare leaflets with additional information for people to take away. These could also be used as summaries for dissemination to people unable to attend a poster session, but who have either had some involvement in the work or have expressed interest in the project.

Summaries for local dissemination

There is always a time lag (rarely less than a year) between completion of a study and the publication of the findings. So, you may wish to prepare summaries of the report for dissemination to individuals who participated in the project, advised or assisted you with the work and/or expressed an interest in the results. It is perhaps only courteous to acknowledge the interest and participation of others (especially those who gave their time and commitment) by keeping them informed of your progress and findings. The level of detail in the summary will depend on the intended audience.

PRESENTING AT A CONFERENCE

Local, national or international conferences are commonly the fora where the wider dissemination of research findings will be commenced. Conferences are usually organised with specific audiences in mind, e.g. they may be principally for researchers or practitioners, professionals from one discipline or across disciplines. The anticipated audience is often an important factor in your selection of a suitable conference. By presenting your work at a conference you can bring your work into the public domain more quickly than by publication in a peer-reviewed journal. Also, you will receive some immediate feedback from, and have an opportunity to discuss your work with, colleagues undertaking similar work or with interests in the same field. This may help you to identify other issues or perspectives surrounding your work. It may also help you to consider how you may approach publication, or plan to follow up your research. Discussion of findings at a conference does not generally preclude the subsequent submission of the research to a journal.

Conferences may be advertised one or even two years in advance, so you may want to be on the look-out for an appropriate forum from the early stages. The first step in presenting your work at a conference is the submission of an abstract. Abstracts will usually have to be submitted to conference organisers around six months before the conference.

Writing a conference abstract

It is on the basis of the abstract that a decision will be made about whether or not to accept your work for presentation at the conference. Abstracts are brief (often one A4 page). Requirements for the structure vary, and it is important that you conform because the abstract, if accepted, may be inserted directly into an abstract book or the conference proceedings.

In writing the abstract it is helpful to follow an introduction, methods, results, discussion structure, even it this is not a requirement. The abstract is effectively a summary of the study prepared with a particular audience in mind. As a result of its brevity, the introduction will often be confined to two or three sentences, although the aims and objectives must be clear. The methods will also be brief but should communicate key information such as type of study (e.g. quantitative or qualitative), study setting, sampling procedure and sample size, and principal methods of data collection, processing and analysis. An overview of the results should be included; however, space will permit only limited detail and this is all that will usually be expected. The abstract should conclude with a comment on the important findings and their implications.

The content of the abstract (and hence the material to be presented at the conference) will be influenced by the conference audience, e.g. the messages and focus of your talk will depend on whether you are addressing a group of researchers, health professionals, students or others.

The selection of abstracts by the conference organisations will frequently follow a refereeing process. The abstracts will be forwarded to members of a scientific committee who will comment on their suitability for presentation at the conference. The criteria used in this assessment are sometimes published in advance, but often include the scientific validity of the research and relevance to the conference themes and audience.

At many conferences research is presented in both oral and poster sessions. You may have the opportunity to express your preference. Some guidance on the choice of oral or poster presentation and their preparation is provided above.

PAPERS FOR PUBLICATION

Publication of their research in a paper is a goal to which researchers aspire. Publication in a relevant journal should be considered for research that provides new information or insights, contains important messages for practitioners, policy-makers or other bodies, and is carried out to a high standard.

The first step is to decide which journal would be most appropriate. If the research was addressing issues relevant to pharmacy practice and the messages were for pharmacists, you could choose a pharmacy journal. If the focus was on other aspects of drug use or clinical practice you might consider an interprofessional or more clinical journal. It is sensible to send the work to a journal where research into similar topic areas has previously been published, because this may be a place that people with an interest in that field expect to find, and therefore regularly look for, recent work. You may also decide whether the study is relevant to a local, national or international audience.

Your decision about where to submit for publication may also be governed by the type of paper you wish to write. Some journals are dedicated to academic research with an emphasis on methodology, whereas others (although still seeing rigour in methodology as important) focus on work that has an explicit application, e.g. relevance to health policy or professional practice. You may decide that, rather than prepare an academic paper, you would prefer to write a more informal article or commentary based on the project and its findings.

A research paper will comprise an abstract, followed by introduction, methods, results and discussion sections. All journals publish 'instructions for authors' which state their more specific requirements. The project report may provide a framework for a paper. However, some restructuring will be required to ensure that the focus of the paper is relevant to the journal's readership and conforms to their house style. Sometimes additional literature work or data analysis will be required.

After submission, it is usual for the paper to undergo peer review. The editor will send copies of the paper to independent researchers, who will be asked to comment on issues such as the subject area of the paper and the originality of the work, the methodological rigour, importance of the findings, validity of the conclusions, suitability for the journal's readership, and whether or not they would recommend publication. The editor will then make a decision on whether or not to accept the paper. The reviewers' comments are sent to the authors. If the paper is accepted it is common for this to be conditional upon some revision in accordance with the suggestions and recommendations of the reviewers. After acceptance for publication, there will often be a delay of several months before the paper appears in print. Before publication, a copy of the proofs is usually sent to the corresponding author for a final check. Publication of research is a protracted process. A year from submission to publication is not untypical.

CONCLUSION

The aspiration of researchers to have their work published in well-respected journals is not misplaced. This is particularly so for pharmacy practice and related research, which is generally undertaken with a particular application in view. Work that remains unpublished is unlikely to contribute to current debates or influence service development. It is unrealistic to expect that many projects that are undertaken as part of an MPharm degree, because of the short time-frame, will lead directly to publication. This work is important, however, in that it commonly contributes to a wider research programme, the outcomes of which will be published. Therefore, it is important that the project is pursued to a high scientific standard and that the report includes the relevant information and detailed discussion that would be required to support a publication.

Further reading

There are numerous texts devoted to health services research methodology, and to produce an exhaustive list would not be feasible. Both for general descriptions of health services research methodology and for more detailed discussions of particular methods and procedures, there will be a wide variety of possible books and journal articles that can be explored and may be very helpful. It may be sensible to start with those that are either recommended by a project supervisor or readily available to you. There are, however, very few texts that are dedicated to the application of health services research methodology specifically in pharmacy settings. The list below provides some suggestions of texts that may be useful in providing further discussion on approaches and methods that are commonly employed in pharmacy practice research.

Bowling A (2002) *Research Methods in Health*, 2nd edn. Milton Keynes: Open University Press.

Bryman A, Burgess RG (eds) (1994) *Analysing Qualitative Data*. London: Routledge.

COREC (Central Office for Research Ethics Committees): www.corec.org.uk.

Florey C du V (1993) Sample size for beginners. *BMJ* 306: 1181–4.

Kirkwood B, Sterne J (2003) *Essential Medical Statistics*. Oxford: Blackwell Sciences.

McConway K, Davey B (eds) (2001) *Studying Health and Disease*. Milton Keynes: Open University Press.

Miles MB, Huberman AM (eds) (1994) *Qualitative Data Analysis: An expanded sourcebook*. London: Sage.

Oppenheim AN (1992) *Questionnaire Design, Interviewing and Attitude Measurement*, 2nd edn. London: Pinter Publishers.

Smith FJ (2002) *Research Methods in Pharmacy Practice*. London: Pharmaceutical Press.

Taylor K, Harding G (eds) (2001) *Pharmacy Practice. Part 7: Research Methods*. London: Taylor & Francis.

Index